# GERD and Acid Reflux

# Diet

# Cookbook

**"Complete guide to prevent, treat GERD and acid reflux with natural remedies."**

**Charles Thompson**

# Copyright© 2020 by Charles Thompson

## All rights reserved.

# Contents

# Acid Reflux Diet Cookbook

## Introduction

Acid reflux is a common digestive condition that creates irritation, heartburn, and pain at the opening of the stomach as well as burning in the food canal. A person experiences this issue due to the reverse flow of the fluid and food from the stomach towards the throat. All over the world, people commonly face acid reflux and other related issues, which can be worse if not treated on time and properly. According to health consultants, the increased ratio of acid reflux issues is due to inappropriate food consumption, poor food options, lack of sleep, stressful mental conditions, and lack of physical activity in people's everyday routine. The digestive system is a sensitive part of the body and can be easily disturbed due to any physical exertion or mental restlessness.

The continuous problem with gastric issues can influence a person's productivity and thinking ability. It can restrict a person's activities and can be the cause of severe ulcer or esophageal cancer as well. the best and most natural way to treat acid reflux and its complications is a change of lifestyle. Following proper diet plans and implementing exercise routines can help a person to overcome the reflux and improve their digestive health. People with obesity, diabetes, or who have inflammation issues can easily be affected by acid reflux. According to doctors, it is recommended that to overcome and avoid the gastric acid reflux, a person should maintain a healthy weight and keep active for at least 30 to 40 minutes at a time on a regular basis.

This book provides enough information about acid reflux, its causes, symptoms and treatment options. As well as for the reader, it has the information that reveals how lifestyle changes can improve a person's overall health and reduce the signs and complications of acid reflux. For those with diet concerns, we have included some healthy and delicious recipes for those who are living with acid reflux. This way, those struggling with this issue can still have or enjoy the delicious food. It has many other interesting and informative facts about acid reflux and how to treat this condition with natural, healthy food.

# Chapter 1: Gastric Acid Reflux

The human body is a complex one that is crafted very well. Everything is connected to each other and all the organs or tissues are working in perfect synchronization. If one thing goes wrong, then it will put a direct effect on the rest of the body as well. Our stomach is one of the integral organs of the body that affects many other parts as well. If your stomach is not working as it should, then your skin will be dull, and you will have acne, scars, heartburn, bloating, pain and a feeling of unrest. Among all these things, you may feel acid reflux in the body.

Acid reflux is a condition of having a burning pain that is similar to heartburn in lower chest or sometimes your food pipe or throat as well. When the stomach acid flows upward to the food pipe, it causes the acidic feeling to the pipe and lower chest. Sometimes in severe conditions is can come up to the throat, cause severe pain, and make you uncomfortable.

It seems to be a commonly experienced feeling by a majority of people in their daily routine, sometimes once in a week and sometimes in every 15 to 20 days. A person is diagnosed with the gastric acid reflux when he or she is experiencing the feeling more than twice a week. In such conditions, it is necessary for the person to move forward and ask for medical help.

## Causes

Before heading for a doctor, it is necessary to look into the causes of acid reflux. Whenever our body is not functioning properly or an organ is behaving differently, there are certain reasons behind that. It is important to identify these reasons and problems in the first place. When you know the causes, you will be able to move toward a better treatment and prevention system. Therefore, here we are, discussing some of the major causes that lead to acid reflux.

### Hiatus or Hernia

One of the non-preventable causes of acid reflux is the Hiatus or Hernia.

It is a condition when a hole occurs in diaphragm that leads to the upper part of the stomach to enter the chest cavity. This situation can cause the acid from stomach to reflux in the upper canal and cause the burning sensation in throat and chest section.

It is one of the critical conditions in overall human health, as the person will not be able to control the factor. Only a surgery and proper treatment to the hernia can help to avoid the gastric acid reflux in such conditions. There is a 100 percent chance of acid reflux in hernia patients, as both sections intersect one other in this situation.

## Obesity

Another cause of gastric acid reflux is obesity. When there is a lack of weight management, then our body behaves differently. Weight that is above average has an intense reaction in the body. Organs start behaving differently and this can result in issues. Obesity is not a normal condition; in fact, it is connected to a number of health risks. Increased weight and body mass affect total body stamina, bone strength, heart performance, blood circulation, hormonal changes and organ activities.

Gastric acid reflux is one of the major outcomes that are related to obesity. The stomach is unable to digest all the food properly, and the acid release is an effort to deal with the excessive energy left in the body. It causes the outward flow of acid from the stomach. Moreover, obesity can affect the stomach size and its movement can trigger the condition of acid reflux.

## Smoking

Smoking is one of the biggest causes of acid reflux. It is a known fact that cigarettes and cigars have acidic reactions in the body. Moreover, smoking affects the overall organ system composition as well. It can not only affect the lungs, but the stomach as well. In response to the smoke and all the chemicals in it, the acid in the stomach reaches the food canal in reverse. When the person inhales and exhales smoke, it can come up with fumes of acid from the stomach and can increase the risks and effects of gastric acid reflux.

## Alcohol

Another major cause of acid reflux is the use of alcohol. Alcoholism is dangerous for a person's overall health. It affects the lifestyle and internal organs of the body. The consumption of alcohol is good if kept within a safe limit, but when there is excessive use, there will be problems. Acid reflux is one of the problems that are caused as a result of excessive alcohol consumption. The important thing is to keep the consumption of alcohol in normal routine and keep it limited for the safe use.

## No or low physical activity

The food we eat is digested in our stomach and the process is triggered by two major things. One is acid, and the other is physical activity. If a person eats and has no or low physical activity, then there can be a chance of acid reflux. The stomach will produce acid in order to digest food, but the excessive amount of acid will produce a reflux in the food canal in the event of no activity. It is important to have a walk after a meal or exert your body physically to trigger the proper digestion of your food. It will help you to make things better and smooth as well. Physical activity will help you to make the better use of acid in the stomach and get it dissolved in the food. It will neutralize the acid in the digestion process and will get you all the necessary nutrients you need.

## Multiple drugs and sedatives

Sometimes the sedative medications and anti-depressant drugs we take can cause acidity in the stomach. That acidity can lead to ultimate gastric acid reflux. It is necessary to have a safe and limited dosage of the drugs. The excessive use of medicine, especially without prescriptions, could affect your overall stomach functions.

## Pregnancy

During pregnancy, there are numerous changes that occur. From mood swings to food options and psychological ideas to physical movements, everything changes. During this process, females have threats to face, many of them being critical health constraints. It can happen sometimes due to lack of care, vitamins, or excessive use of a specific product. There are sometimes the genetic reactions in the body as well. Acid reflux is something that is not inherited, but it can be caused by pregnancy and body changes. Your stomach may behave differently and you may not be getting as physical movement, so it can lead to a reflux situation.

Moreover, the vomiting and constant nausea caused by pregnancy can always trigger the gastric acid reflux. In this regard, the important thing is to monitor everything and then have essential solutions.

## Poor dietary selection

Your food intake and dietary choices matter a lot when it comes to your overall health. Acid reflux can be triggered by poor dietary options. If you are consuming junk food, soft drinks, dried snacks, and fat rich food options then you may feel the hits of acid reflux. Such food options increase the acidity in the stomach and can result in issues.

## Improper posture after meal

Acid reflux is not just caused by medical deficiencies and complications. In fact, it can come up as a reaction to bad posture . It is necessary to ensure the proper physical posture when having meal. Bending over your waist or lying on your back while eating or right after taking meal can result in acid reflux. It can be dangerous and build up the issue for more serious causes. It is necessary to watch out during your meal and pay attention to your movement routine in order to avoid such drastic outcomes from your activities.

### Bedtime snacks

Bedtime snacking is one of the common habits that people have. It is a kind of regular routine for people in many cases. On the other hand, it is one of the critical causes of acid reflux. Eating food at bedtime does not allow it to digest properly, and the physical posture that often accompanies bedtime snacking can cause the stomach acids to reflux upwards.

## Symptoms

Most people confuse gastric acid reflux with heartburn. Sometimes it is claimed that both are same and sometimes they are marked as different. Although there is a fine line difference between the two, it is necessary to underline the difference focusing on the symptoms of acid reflux. You can fight with a medical condition after knowing its causes and major symptoms. The symptoms are necessary for the better evaluation and diagnosis.

Acid reflux is one of the conditions that people do not take seriously in the beginning. Lately, when things are a bit out of control, they became concerned about the issue. In order to live healthily, the important thing is to keep the symptoms and all changes in the body under consideration. It is good to know the major symptoms and take note of these symptoms. Eventually, it will help in self and early diagnosis and then you can come up with the best of remedies and treatments. Here are a few major symptoms of gastric acid reflux to consider:

- Heartburn is one of the major symptoms of acid reflux. It is not the same thing, but the first step that leads to the condition. You can feel a discomfort or pain with a burning sensation in your abdomen and chest area that goes up to your throat.
- Bitter tasting in back side of mouth and throat is another symptom that is shows the bad stomach condition and acid reflux
- Burning sensation in the upper throat can be a reaction of acid reflux

- You can feel nausea and an ultimate feeling of throwing up the food you just had
- Continuous burping with a bad smell and acidic feeling
- Vomit can be bloody and painful in severe cases
- Acid reflux can cause black and bloody stools, accompanied by a burning sensation
- There can be difficult hiccups with a mixed feeling of pain and burning
- The immense reduction in weight can be observed without any reason
- Sore throat, dry cough, and wheezing can occur in initial and chronic stages of acid reflux
- There can be a feeling of unease in the throat, like food is stuck in the throat and will be out in no time
- Difficulty in swallowing food, with pain and burning
- Bad breath and dental erosion are other major symptoms of acid reflux

The condition of acid reflux not only affects the stomach and causes a burning sensation inside. In fact, it leads to some major outcomes. If there is not proper treatment of the condition, then results can be drastic. It can start as a simple problem of indigestion or acidity in the stomach that will lead to burping and even up resulting in bloody vomit, difficulty in swallowing and much more. It is necessary to identify these basic symptoms initially and take measures in order to resolve these issues quickly.

You can get to know more symptoms of acid reflux in certain cases. It is not necessary that everyone will face the same issues in the beginning. The person could have any of these or all of these symptoms from time to time. The best way is to be alert with the treatment, even if you are facing the initial or minor symptoms. Sometimes you may have these issues mixed with any other health condition, then make sure to discuss this with your physician in the first place.

Remember, bad smell and throat issues largely come from your stomach, and if these go unnoticed, then you may have to face the music. Note the symptoms and related symbols of the problem and consider these things in your daily routine for early diagnosis and control of the problem.

# Treatments

Gastric acid reflux seems to be a common and normal issue. However, in extreme cases,, it can be lethal. If you are ignoring the condition and not concerned about getting treatment, you will still have to face the issues in the end. Whenever a person is suffering from the acid reflux, it is necessary to go for the treatment and remedies in the first place. Without a proper and organized treatment, it is not possible to recover from the condition, and it can cause issues in the long run. Here are some treatment options that one could consider.

## Medications

During the initial stage when a person is facing issues with heartburn or acidity, there are certain medications to use to control these symptoms. It is necessary to use these medications after the proper consultation. Remember you may mix up heartburn and acid reflux with each other. Heartburn can be a condition in acid reflux, but it is not the acid reflux all the time.

Gaviscon is one of the famous and commonly used drugs to treat problems related to heartburn. It is one of the mild and effective sources that help to reduce the burning in the initial scale. If you have the severe case of acid reflux, then you will get the drugs in combination of famotidine, ranitidine, cimetidine, rebeprazole, omeprazole and others. Make sure to consult a physician in severe cases for the medication prescription and keep up with regular checkups.

## Surgery

When it is not possible to treat the condition of acid reflux using medications, then doctors have another option: surgery. To treat conditions, there are two types of surgeries depending on the condition and the patient's situation. In the first type of surgical procedure, there is a placement of a LINX device around and outside the lowered end of the esophagus or food pipe. The device is made of titanium wires that work as a barrier to fluid flowing outward from the stomach. The device helps patients to quit or reduce medication intake. Having the device after a surgery comes with a number of limitations. For example, the patient can never have MRI test later on. Moreover, it is necessary to check if the patient is allergic to any metal or not.

The second surgical procedure is the fundoplication that helps to reduce the acid reflux. In the procedure, an artificial valve is attached to the top of stomach that wraps the upper part of the stomach and reduces the chances of acid reflux. It can be a treatment for the hiatal hernia as well.

Both of these surgical procedures should be considered a last resort in the case of acid reflux. The first preference in every case is prevention using lifestyle changes, the second is medication with major lifestyle changes. In the end, if the condition is critical and patient needs ultimate help, then surgery is the option that doctors should eventually resort to.

## Lifestyle

Along with the medication or surgery when you are suffering from acid reflux, then you need to make some essential lifestyle changes. Adopting some of the right habits and making a difference in your routine will help you to be good and better with the treatment. Here are the major changes you need to make in your daily routine:

- Take a light and spice free diet
- Eat healthy and fresh
- Eat in intervals
- Take your medications on time
- Do not wear tight clothes or belts

- Take your meals in intervals and in small portions
- Increase your physical activity to help your body consume energy and reduce weight if you are overweight

## Risks and Complications

If there is a lack of concern towards the issue and you delay treatment, then it can lead to some drastic complications. They can seem to be minor issues, but can never be so reckless that you must face the critical music. Here are the complications you may have to face:

- The borderline of the esophagus can be damaged and inflamed, causing constant irritation, internal bleeding, and ulceration in some cases.
- There can be a non-stop burning and internal irritation that can affect the overall health and enhance psychological pressure as well.
- There can be scar development that will lead to difficult swallowing and food will not be able to travel down the esophagus
- The repeated exposure of the cells and tissues to the stomach acid can change their formation. It can damage the cell structure, causing them to be dead and potentially leading to cancer development.

It is necessary to focus on the problem in the first stage in order to help with the proper treatment. In case of permanent negligence, things can be difficult to control and will come up with some of the ultimately damaging results as a whole.

# Chapter 2: Prevention of Acid Reflux

Prevention is better than treatment, as we all know. It is not just a phrase but in all matters, it is the ultimate solution and escape. No matter from what disease you are going through, you need to make sure that you will adopt some of the important preventions that will help you to live a healthy life.

In case of acid reflux, things are quite manageable and in your hand. There are certain preventions that help to keep your body in order. It is not something that is caused by any external virus or infection; it is all about the mismanagement in your daily routine. With a little management and care, you can stop or revert things in the initial stage. It is quite easy to follow the prevention guide for acid reflux.

What are some common preventions?

The preventions for acid reflux are more related to your food options than hygienic conditions. It is a kind of lifestyle problem that can occur and trigger to your mismanagement with food, posture, habits, and lifestyle as well. Therefore, it is necessary that you follow some safe lifestyle options in order to avoid further damage to your body.

Using the prevention options, you will be able to avoid the factors that can cause acid reflux, such as heartburn, obesity, depression, drugs, hernia and much more. In our body, everything is linked with each other and you have to make sure that your overall body is healthy. Overall health is something that can help you to be good in life and avoid all the serious threats and issues.

## How Does Food Help?

All problems related to stomach are directly connected to food. The food or diet we use is one of the integral factors in our body. All the minerals and nutrients we get from our food helps us to grow. In case if we do not eat properly or have the right food that we need, it means we can have some deficiencies in the body as well. From the beginning of our lives, cycle doctors recommend having the best food and diet plan in general. There should be everything healthy and well-composed in terms of nutrition, so the body will not have any deficiencies at all.

We once took care of everything in the diet since the birth of a child. Other supplements for nutrition are for emergency use when only diet is not helping the situation. Therefore, in order to prevent acid reflux, we need to get help from food in the first place. It is one of the best resources that will help you throughout life to manage the symptoms of acid reflux. If you want to avoid acid reflux, food helps. If you want to treat acid reflux during the initial stage, food helps. If you have undergone surgery and are trying to maintain your condition, food helps. In short, no matter what your condition is, food is the factor that actually helps you to keep things in control. The question is how it can help you and what you can get out of it.

In order to prevent acid reflux using food therapy, it is necessary to make a food selection that helps you in the following manner:

## Reduce acidity

It is necessary to eat food that reduces acidity and that does not have an acidic nature. As such, you cannot take coffee, alcohol, citrus and other foods that increase the acidic ratio in stomach. By taking the food that reduces acidity and that is lighter in nature, this will help your stomach to be better and reduce its acidic fluency. Moreover, it will not let the acid to reflux in the food pipe or cause burning in the stomach.

## Provide the best nutrients

When you are recovering from acid reflux, your stomach is weak and it affects your overall body as well. You need to choose the food options with the best nutrients. Make sure to eat healthy food enriched with calcium, magnesium and phosphorus. Fruits like bananas, apples and berries help to reduce acidity. Make sure to avoid the processed food with many spices that can kill the nutrients in the food.

## Reduce inflammation

Inflammation or burning is primarily caused by the unlimited spices and sauces we use in our food. It is necessary to take mild spices and sauces in order to keep your dietary choices light. The food spices can increase the burning sensation and double up the inflammation as well. You need to pick up food options with minimum spices or no spices in certain conditions. Moreover, choose to have anti-inflammatory food options that will help you to reduce the overall inflammation in the organs and body.

## Helps to repair organs

There are food options like meat, white meat, grains, and sprouts that are enriched with protein and have the nature to repair body cells internally. The continuous acid reflux in the body causes the organs and cells to become damaged at a large scale. You need some extra nutrients to ensure the proper recovery of these cells and to have better health overall. In this manner, you need to pick up the food options that help in cell repairing and that makes you feel better from the inside out. It will be an overall benefit for you.

## Keep the digestion process lighter

Some major issues with the acid reflux are with digestion. The acid in the stomach is produced to digest food when we eat so much acidic food that the acid's ratio gets higher and causes a reflux. In order to avoid such conditions, it is necessary to eat food that is lighter to digest. It will help the stomach to produce a lesser amount of acid and digest the food easily. Moreover, the food will not be acidic in nature so it will get mixed in the stomach acid and neutralize the overall equation. It is a little science but overall helps to avoid any critical condition that will make you suffer in future on a larger scale.

The best food options to reduce and prevent acid reflux

Not all healthy diet plans or food options are effective enough to help you with the acid reflux prevention and treatment. You need to pick up the specific combinations and safe food options that help to reduce inflammation, burning and acidity. Moreover, you need to keep a balance between your food intake so things will be balanced and work appropriately. Here are some major food options that you can use to prevent acid reflux or to have a quick recovery from the problem:

- Fresh vegetables that are rich in nutrients and low in fat and sugar
- Ginger
- Non-citrus fruits like banana, guava, apple, kiwi and more
- Lean meat and sea food
- Healthy fats like coconut oil, organic butter and more
- Egg whites

All these foods are not acidic in nature and reduce fats from the body. It is a good option to treat these foods as a priority. They can help in prevention and quick recovery from the acid reflux at the beginning. On the other hand, it's important to take a healthy diet seriously so that you can help your body to increase immunity and fight back these issues and problems.

## Lifestyle Changes

In order to prevent acid reflux and have a quick recovery, in addition to controlling your diet, you need to make some lifestyle changes. These changes help bring about quick and effective recovery as well as prevention from the problem. These changes not only help to avoid the acid reflux problem but to have a better life and avoid any further health constraints.

### Eat healthy

In your lifestyle changes, the very first thing you need to do is to eat healthy food. Even if you are eating processed meals, refined sugar, and other things, then make sure to substitute them with healthier alternatives. There should be an irregular pattern of the consumption of these food options. You need to make healthy food options your priority in order to avoid such issues and complications.

## Plan your meals

Make sure to take your meals on time at specific intervals. Eating too much or having meals with long breaks in between can never be healthy. You need to feed your stomach with a small meal after a specific interval so there will be no acidity in there. The planned interval based meals will help you in the path toward safe digestion.

## Get 8 hours of sleep

Sleep is important to let your food digest and your stomach to work efficiently. Make sure that you are taking healthy and good sleep for 8 hours each night. It should be a quality night of sleep for a continuous 8 hours, not in breaks or parts. In the case of a partial sleep cycle, you will feel more exhausted and drained in the end.

## Manage your stress

Stress and anxiety can actually affect the digestion system of your stomach. It is not ideal for a healthy living if you keep stressing out your body. Make sure that you keep a balance between work life and leisure time in order to relax yourself and avoid any health complications. A stressful brain affects the overall body functions and can cause acid reflux.

## Maintain a balance between food options

Lifestyle changes are not about quitting the food options and limiting yourself to a specific kind of diet. It is about balancing your food options. You need to keep the balance between the food options you want to have and that you can have. Make sure that you pick up the right options that will help you to maintain a good balance in your overall intake.

Do not sleep immediately after meals

It is not an ideal habit to sleep or lay down immediately after having a meal. In such conditions, it is not possible for the stomach to digest the food properly. It increases the chances of acid reflux and acidity in stomach to a maximum level.

### Increase physical exertion

Laziness and being in one place for extended periods of time is one of the triggers for acid reflux. If you are not having good physical activity in your daily routine, that means you are not letting your energy get consumed. In such a situation, the stomach acid stays in the stomach and is not be able to dissolve properly. This can cause refluxes later on. With the help of physical exertion, you will be able to reduce your weight and the chances of acid reflux.

## Impact of Exercise

In the prevention and basic treatment, along with food, lifestyle changes and exercise will have a great impact on your overall results. Exercise and good physical activity can help your body to avoid many complications. Exercise activates all your organs, muscles and tissues. It allows you to consume all the energy taken from the food. Moreover, the stomach will digest the food instantly and the acid will not stay in your stomach later on.

### Lean muscles

By reducing the amount of fats you intake, you have more chances of living a healthy life. In order to be happy and stress free from any issues such as acid reflux, you need to have a healthy body. Regular exercise helps you to have the lean muscles that mean you will have less fats and other related problems. It will also reduce the chances of acidity in your body and allow you to consume all the energy from the food you consume food. Eventually, you can avoid many of the issues and problems related to acid reflux and other related problems.

## Better organ functioning

When our body is in a resting position, it is not possible for all the organs to work efficiently. In the rest position or daily normal routine, not all your organs get the pressure and involved in the physical exertion. It causes these organs to have fats and face issues that can lead to some complications like acid reflux. Our stomach causes acid reflux because our stomach does not get the real word to do because of our inactivity. With the help of continuous efforts and activity, things can be better and you can avoid such problems.

## Weight reduction

Obesity is one of the causes that triggers acid reflux. Workout and exercise not only helps keep your body healthy, but helps to reduce weight as well. It melts down all the fat from the body and gives you all good muscles and only muscular weight. On the other hand, it will help you to get better in the overall health scale so that you can enjoy your life.

## Reduced inflammation

Exercise helps to break and make muscles and cells as well. The exertion activates the repairing muscles in the body that helps to reduce the internal and external inflammation. The acid reflux causes worse inflammation internally and makes the person unrestful. Exercise helps to deal with this painful condition and triggers the body to repair cells and damaged organs.

## Active mind and healthy body

Along with food management, a good exercise routine is a perfect combination for a healthy body and active mind. By working out, you will consume all the excessive energy from the your food. Moreover it will release the stress and tension you have. In the end, you can have an active and peaceful mind with a lighter body. With all the exertion, our brain releases the stress hormones and eliminates them from the body in many ways.

# Chapter 3: Treatment & Complications

Gastric acid reflux is not a chronic disease and people usually feel reflux after having a certain food. It is normal in several cases and can be eliminated and reduced with certain medical or natural remedies. But if it is not treated well or a person is having some digestive system problem, the problem can be persistent and become worse. The chronic disease of acid reflux refers to gastroesophageal reflux diseases. It usually occurs when a person constantly feels acid or food between the canal tube that is linked between the stomach and throat. It is also known as heartburn and creates discomfort and other potential risks to a person's health. In this scenario, a person feels or experiences the undigested food or stomach content in the food tube and to the throat. It can damage the inner lining of the tube and of the stomach walls as well.

Acid reflux quickly influences the people having any other health complications. For example, it is common in those with both type 1 and type 2 diabetes. People with asthma may also suffer from acid reflux. Poor digestion problems or other stomach related diseases can also create acid reflux. The treatment of this problem is necessary to be done on time to overcome other health complications, and if not done, then this can cause multiple serious consequences.

According to research, it is shown that acid reflux can be due to improper food intake and consumption of too much fried food and carbonated drinks. This can weaken the power of the stomach to easily digest the food and it can become reactive towards it. Sometimes other health problems can be behind gastric acid reflux. But during the initial stages, with the little concentration of food intake and lifestyle changes, the problem can easily be treated and overcome before it becomes a significant problem.

## Treatment of Acid Reflux

Due to poor lifestyle and unhealthy routine, this leads to different health problems, and acid reflux is one of them. Our lives are too much occupied, even that it is hard to find time to eat at the right time. This increases bad food choices and leads to inappropriate meal times. This increases the weight of a person and can lead to obesity. These activities directly impact your sleep and mind activity. When a person does not have a sound mind and feels restless, the digestive system is the most sensitive part of the whole body. This system feels the effects of the stress first.. This leads to inappropriate food digestion and increases acid reflux.

According to the doctors and health advisors, acid reflux is a treatable problem, and with some lifestyle changes, it can be overcome easily. In the treatment of acid reflux, the first thing that matters is diagnosis. In the first recommendation, food that is not allowed to consume includes: fried and fatty food items, processed and canned food, carbonated drinks, alcoholic drinks, citrus, and pepper. These foods can increase the heartburn and restless condition and can create irritation or damage.

Other than the food restriction, it is necessary to reduce the size of the meal that a person consumes in a day. A large meal size can fill the stomach and increase the reaction or irritation. But with smaller meal sizes, the stomach can have a large space and as a result, this reduces the refluxes. As well as it is necessary to take the last meal 3 hours before going to sleep, and do not consume food right before bedtime.

To neutralize the condition, keep your head parallel to the body when you are on the bed. It helps to control the flow of food or acid towards the food canal and offer relieve for heartburn at nighttime. Do not use a high pillow, because it puts exertion or pressure on the stomach and can create a restless condition.

With the lifestyle and dietary changes implemented, keep consulting the doctor and get medication as well. The medication can help to neutralize the impact and prevent the acid reflux from gaining a serious impact on your health.

## Complications Due to Acid Reflux

Acid reflux is a digestive related problem that can be treated with the medication and a change in lifestyle. But if not treated properly and if the condition is allowed to go untreated for a long time, then it can affect the stomach and other body parts as well. It is reflux or backflow of stomach acid or food towards the food canal that creates heartburn. Due to the movement of the fluid in the throat, a person may experience irritation and dry cough as well. A person with gastric acid reflux usually feels the pain in the chest that feels like a heart pain, but it is actually due to the gas and the effect of reflux comes from the stomach.

Sometimes the symptoms get worse if not treated on time. Acid reflux can damage the inner lining of the esophagus or can be a reason for bleeding as well. This complication can create a stomach ulcer or can be chronic with time. Due to untreated stomach acid reflux, it is also noticed that some people even face the chronic problem of narrowing of their esophagus lining. With time, it can be the cause of esophageal cancer as well. This severe complication cannot just affect the person's health but also can be the cause of limited activities or reduced productivity. In the worst scenario, these can be life-threatening as well.

The best remedy to avoid such issues is to keep the focus on a small problem and get the proper treatment from the health advisor on time.

If you are at the initial stage or facing the acid reflux, then it is important to pay attention to your activities. With just small change in their diet and lifestyle, a person cannot just overcome the issue but also get the treatment they need on time. Even with natural food and home-based remedies, it is easy to treat and control acid reflux. All you need is to avoid the unhealthy or acidic food choices that increase the acidity in the stomach. Consume the food with minimum spices and salt that reduces the irritation. Also have small meal sizes throughout the day. Furthermore, we have some recipes that will help you to make delicious food that offers relief for acid reflux as well.

# Chapter 4: Recipes for Breakfast

### 1. Soft & delicious French toast
*Preparation time*: 10 minutes | *Cooking time*: 08 minutes | *Servings*: 4

**Ingredients:**

- 4 eggs
- 1 ½ teaspoons crushed cinnamon
- 1 teaspoon vanilla extract
- A pinch of salt

- 8 slices of sandwich bread
- ¾ cup milk
- 2 tablespoon ground sugar
- 1 tablespoon butter

**Directions:**

In a bowl, whisk eggs well. Add vanilla extract, salt, and milk. Mix all the ingredients well. Dip the bread slices in the egg mixture. Take another bowl and mix cinnamon and sugar together. Now sprinkle this ground sugar and cinnamon on both sides of the bread. Take a nonstick pan with butter. Heat the butter and cook the egg soaked slices until its color becomes golden brown. Cook it for 3 to 4 minutes per side on a low medium flame. Serve and enjoy.

**Nutritional Information:** Carbohydrates 39g, Calories 370, Protein 14g, Fats: 17g, Sugar 9g.

2. **Cinnamon & vanilla toast**
   ***Preparation time****: 5 minutes | **Cooking time***: 5 minutes |
   ***Servings****: 2*

## Ingredients:

- 3 eggs
- 1 tablespoon butter
- 1 teaspoon vanilla extract
- A pinch of sugar
- 5 slices sandwich bread
- 3 tablespoons milk
- A pinch of salt
- ½ teaspoon cinnamon

## Directions:

Take a bowl and mix eggs, milk, salt, sugar, cinnamon, and vanilla extract together. Whisk all the ingredients well. Soak the bread slices in the mixture properly. Now take a skillet with the butter and place it over a medium-low flame. Once the butter is melted, place the slices in the skillet one by one to cook. Cook it for around two to three minutes on each sides and it is ready to serve. If you want, you can also serve it with the maple syrup, but this is optional.

**Nutritional Information:** Carbohydrates 51g, Calories 422, Protein 8g, Fats: 16g, Sugar 18g.

3. **Breakfast frittata**
   ***Preparation time****: 15 minutes | **Cooking time***: 15 minutes |
   ***Servings****: 8*

## Ingredients:

- 3 tablespoons chopped onions
- 1 cup cubed boiled potatoes
- 1 cup ground cooked sausage
- ¼ cup sliced tomatoes
- 12 eggs
- 2 tablespoons finely chopped parsley

- 2 tablespoons olive oil
- ½ cup grated cheese
- ½ teaspoon black pepper
- ½ cup ground bacon
- 1 teaspoon salt

**Directions:**

Place the oven skillet over a medium flame. Add oil and add potatoes and onion in it and cook for around 5 minutes. Now add tomatoes, sausage, and bacon and cook for a minute. In a bowl, beat the eggs, salt, and black pepper. Now carefully pour the beaten eggs into the pan. Cook it for few minutes and when it's more than half cooked, add cheese and parsley in it. Now put the skillet in the oven to cook it for around 10 minutes in the preheated oven at a temperature of 350F.

**Nutritional Information:** Carbohydrates 05g, Calories 268, Protein 16g, Fats: 20g, Sugar 1g.

4. **Scrambled egg with veggies**
   **Preparation time**: 5 minutes I **Cooking time**: 10 minutes I
   **Servings**: 2

**Ingredients:**

- 4 eggs
- ¼ cup milk

- ½ teaspoon salt
- 1/8 teaspoon black pepper
- ½ cup cubed mushrooms

- 1 chopped tomatoes
- ½ cup ground green pepper

- ¼ cup cubed green onions
- ½ cup grated broccoli

**Directions:**

Take a medium-sized mixing bowl and mix egg, milk, green pepper, black pepper, salt, and onion in it. Mix the ingredients well until all the ingredients are well blended. Take a pan and cook the mushrooms and broccoli for around 5 minutes. Add spinach and cook for an additional 2 minutes. Now add the prepared mixture. Now add tomatoes and cook the eggs properly for around 3 to 4 minutes. Transfer it to the serving plate. The scrambled eggs and veggies are ready to serve.

**Nutritional Information:** Carbohydrates 9g, Calories 96, Protein 14g, Fats 10g, Sugar 4g.

### 5. Eggs benedict
***Preparation time***: 10 minutes I ***Cooking time***: 20 minutes I ***Servings***: 4

**Ingredients:**

- 4 eggs
- 4 bacon slices
- 1 tablespoon lemon juice
- ½ cup melted butter
- 2 egg yolks

- 1 tablespoon warm water
- 1 tablespoon butter
- 2 split and toasted muffins
- A pinch salt

**Directions:**

Place water filled pan over the high flame and bring it to boil. Now reduce the flame and break an egg gently in a bowl and gently transfer it to the pan. Cook them for around 3 minutes. Now, with the help of a spatula, transfer the eggs from the pan to a paper towel. In a skillet, melt the butter over a medium-high flame. Now cook bacon in this butter for around 4 minutes. Place the bacon on the first half of the muffin and place cooked eggs on it. To make the sauce, add egg yolks, lemon juice, salt, pepper, and water in a blender and blend it thoroughly. Add hot melted butter and blend it well. Now pour the sauce on the muffins over eggs and serve.

**Nutritional Information:** Carbohydrates 29.6g, Calories 879, Protein 31.8g, Fats: 71.1g.

6. **Pear banana nut muffins**

*Preparation time*: 5 minutes I ***Cooking time***: 15 minutes I
***Servings***: 12

## Ingredients:

- ½ cup crumbled almonds
- 1 peeled and ground pear
- ¾ cup milk
- 2 cups flour
- 1 teaspoon vanilla
- ½ cup rolled oats
- 2 mashed bananas
- 1 teaspoon cinnamon
- ½ cup melted coconut oil

## Directions:

Preheat the oven to 360F. Set the 24 muffin cups in a baking tray and
prepare them with the baking sheet. Set these cups aside. Now take a
big mixing bowl and add all the ingredients in it. Whisk all the
ingredients well and pour the mixture in the prepared muffin cups
evenly. Bake the muffins for 15 minutes. Check them by inserting a
matchstick in the middle and bake the muffins until the match stick
comes out clean. At this point, the muffins are ready to serve.

**Nutritional Information:** Carbohydrates 13g, Calories 119, Protein 2g,
Fats: 6g, Sugar 2g.

7. **Blueberry muffins**

*Preparation time*: 10 minutes I ***Cooking time***: 30 minutes I
***Servings***: 12

## Ingredients:

- 2 cups flour
- ½ cup milk
- 2 teaspoons baking powder
- 1 ¼ cups sugar
- ½ teaspoon salt
- 2 eggs
- ½ cup butter
- 2 cups washed and drained blueberries
- 1 teaspoon vanilla extract
- 3 teaspoons sugar

## Directions:

In a bowl, mix butter and 1 ½ cup sugar well. Now add eggs and vanilla extract and whisk them well. Now add all the remaining ingredients in this batter and whisk it well until all the ingredients are merged properly. Take a baking dish and set the 12 muffin cups in the baking dish with the muffin liner. Now pour the batter in the prepared cups and sprinkle the sugar on tops. Place the cups in the preheated oven at 375F for around 30 to 35 minutes or until baked well.

**Nutritional Information:** Carbohydrates 39g, Calories 252, Protein 4g, Fats: 9g, Sugar 22g.

## 8. Pumpkin nut muffins
*Preparation time*: 10 minutes I ***Cooking time***: 10 minutes I *Servings*: 16

**Ingredients:**

- 2 eggs
- 1 cup brown sugar
- 1 ½ teaspoons baking powder
- 1 teaspoon vanilla extract
- 1 cup walnuts
- ½ teaspoon pumpkin pie spice
- 2 cups flour
- ¼ teaspoon cinnamon
- 1 cup melted butter
- ½ teaspoon salt
- 15-ounce pumpkin puree

**Directions:**

Set the oven to 375F and set a tray with muffin cups. Prepare the muffin cups with a baking sheet. Take a bowl and mix baking powder, flour, and salt together. Beat the brown sugar and pumpkin puree in a bowl. Combine eggs, vanilla, and melted butter and whisk well. Now add dry ingredients mixture, walnuts, and remaining ingredients and combine them well. Scoop the prepared batter in the muffin cups evenly. Now place it in the preheated oven to cook for around 18 minutes and it is ready to serve.

**Nutritional Information:** Carbohydrates 27.7g, Calories 122, Protein 3.1g, Fats: 3.3g, Sugar 18.9g.

### 9. Egg & vegetable mix muffin

*Preparation time*: 20 minutes I *Cooking time*: 30 minutes I *Servings*: 4

**Ingredients:**

- 8 eggs
- 2 minced garlic cloves
- 10 sliced mushrooms
- A pinch salt
- 1 tablespoon butter
- 1 chopped onion
- 2 diced bell peppers
- 2 cups chopped spinach
- ½ teaspoon ground black pepper

**Directions:**

Place the skillet over the medium flame and melt the butter. Stir the garlic, bell peppers, and onion in it and cook for around 5 minutes. Add spinach and mushrooms in it and cook for an additional 3 minutes. Add salt and black pepper in it. In a mixing bowl beat the eggs and add the cooked mixture in it. Take the prepared muffin cups with the baking sheet. Pour the batter in the muffin cups and cook them in the preheated oven for around 20 to 25 minutes.

**Nutritional Information:** Carbohydrates 7g, Calories 370, Protein 15g, Fats: 10g.

### 9. Cauliflower breakfast muffin

*Preparation time*: 10 minutes I *Cooking time*: 30 minutes I *Servings*: 6

**Ingredients:**

- 2 eggs
- 2 cups shredded cheese
- 1 tablespoon chopped flaxseed
- ¼ teaspoon salt
- 2 ½ cups cubed cauliflower
- 2/3 cup cubed lean ham
- 1/8 teaspoon ground black pepper

## Directions:

Set the oven at a temperature of 375F. Set 12 muffin cups in a tray with the muffin liner. Take a bowl and beat eggs well. Now add all the remaining ingredients in the eggs and whisk well until all the ingredients are merged well. Spoon the prepared batter in the muffin tins and place them in the preheated oven to bake for around 30 minutes. To check whether it is cooked well, take a match stick and insert it in the middle of a muffin cup. If it comes out clean, it means muffins are ready.

**Nutritional Information:** Carbohydrates 5g, Calories 214, Protein 15g, Fats: 15g, Sugar 2g.

### 10. Carrot & apple oat muffin
*Preparation time*: 15 minutes I *Cooking time*: 25 minutes I *Servings*: 12

## Ingredients:

- 2 eggs
- ½ cup brown sugar
- ½ cup ground sugar
- 1 peeled and ground apple
- 1 cup grated carrots
- 1 cup dried cranberry
- ½ cup olive oil
- ¾ cup oats
- 2 teaspoons vanilla
- ½ cup flour
- 1 teaspoon baking powder
- ½ teaspoon salt

## Directions:

Prepare the muffin cups with the muffin liner and preheat the oven at the temperature of 350F. In a bowl, beat the eggs, vanilla, oil, and sugar well. Now combine oats, baking powder, salt, and flour together and whisk well. In this mixture, add all the remaining ingredients and combine them well. Now pour the mixture in the muffin tins and bake it for around 30 minutes. Leave them for around 5 minutes to cool down and serve.

**Nutritional Information:** Carbohydrates 35g, Calories 281, Protein 11g, Fats: 12g.

## 11. Breakfast egg muffins

*Preparation time*: 5 minutes | *Cooking time*: 20 minutes | *Servings*: 12

**Ingredients:**

- 10 eggs
- ¼ teaspoon ground black pepper
- 1 tablespoon minced fresh chives
- 6 oz. cooked bacon
- ¼ teaspoon salt
- 1/3 cup milk
- 1 cup shredded cheddar cheese

**Directions:**

Set the oven temperature to 375F. Set the 12 muffin tins in a baking dish and place the muffin liner in it. In a mixing bowl, add milk and eggs and beat them well. Now add ¾ cup cheese, salt, pepper, and cooked bacon and mix all the ingredients well. Spoon the mixture in the prepared muffin tins and sprinkle chives and remaining cheese on it. Bake the muffins in the preheated oven for about 20 minutes. Leave them for a few minutes to cool down and then transfer it to the serving plate.

**Nutritional Information:** Carbohydrates 1g, Calories 171, Protein 13g, Fats: 12g.

### 12. Potato & spinach frittata

*Preparation time*: 10 minutes I *Cooking time*: 20 minutes I *Servings*: 6

**Ingredients:**

- 6 eggs
- 1/3 cup milk
- 2 tablespoons cubed onion
- ½ cup grated cheese
- 1/8 ground black pepper

- 6 sliced potatoes
- 2 tablespoons olive oil
- 1 teaspoon minced garlic
- 1 cup roughly chopped spinach
- ½ teaspoon salt

**Directions:**

Place a skillet with olive oil over a medium flame. Add potatoes, cover and cook it for approximately 10 minutes. Add onions, garlic, salt and pepper, and spinach in it and stir for about 2 minutes. Take a mixing bowl and add milk and egg in it and beat them well. Pour the beaten eggs in the skillet of vegetables and reduce the heat. Now add cheddar cheese, cover it with a lid, and cook it for about 5 to 7 minutes.

**Nutritional Information:** Carbohydrates 28g, Calories 281, Protein 12g, Fats: 13g, Sugar 3g.

### 13. Tomato toast with Ricotta

*Preparation time*: 5 minutes I *Cooking time*: 5 minutes I
*Servings*: 4

**Ingredients:**

- 2 tablespoons chopped onion
- 1/8 teaspoon crushed black pepper
- 4 slices of bread
- 1 cup ricotta cheese
- 3 thickly sliced tomatoes
- ¾ teaspoon Italian seasoning

**Directions:**

Take a mixing bowl and combine chopped onion, ricotta cheese, black pepper, and Italian seasoning. Mix until all the ingredients are combined well. Now put this mixture aside. Take the bread slices and toast both sides. It's time to assemble the toast. Take the bread slice and spread the prepared mixture on it. Now, place the tomato slices on it. Now your delicious tomato toast with ricotta is ready to serve.

**Nutritional Information:** Carbohydrates 41g, Calories 127, Protein 12g, Fats: 10g, Sugar 4g.

### 14. Avocado & egg toast

*Preparation time*: 5 minutes I *Cooking time*: 5 minutes I
*Servings*: -1

**Ingredients:**

- 1 egg
- 1 oz. mashed avocado
- A pinch of black pepper
- 1 teaspoon hot sauce
- 1 slice of bread
- A pinch of salt
- 1 tablespoon olive oil

**Directions:**

In a bowl, add the mashed avocado, salt, and pepper together. Mix it well. Take a small non-stick pan and place it over a medium-low flame. Now pour oil in it and carefully crack the egg in the small pan. Cover the pan with its lid and cook it for few minutes. On the other hand, toast the slice and add the mashed avocado on top. Sprinkle salt and pepper on it and place the cooked egg on top. Pour hot sauce over it and serve. Hot sauce is exceptional, so if you wish to add it, you can add it.

**Nutritional Information:** Carbohydrates 23g, Calories 299, Protein 12g, Fats: 10g, Sugar 4g.

### 15. Yogurt & blueberry smoothie
*Preparation time: 5 minutes | Cooking time: 0 minutes | Servings: 3*

**Ingredients:**

- ½ cup yogurt
- 1 sliced banana

- 1 tablespoon ground flaxseed
- A few coconut flakes

- ¾ cup of coconut water
- 2 ½ cups frozen blueberries
- 1 cup baby spinach

- ¼ teaspoon vanilla extract

**Directions:**

Take a blender and combine yogurt, banana, frozen blueberries, spinach, flaxseed, vanilla extract, and coconut water. Blend all the ingredients for about one minute or until the ingredients become the consistency of a smoothie. Add ice in it to chill. If the mixture is thicker and not according to your own desire, add more coconut water or ice to your preference. When the mixture meets your preferred consistency, pour it in the serving glass. Add few coconut flakes as a garnish and serve it immediately.

**Nutritional Information:** Carbohydrates 34g, Calories 180, Protein 9g, Fats: 3g, Sugar 21g.

### 16. Peanut butter & banana smoothie
***Preparation time:*** *5 minutes |* ***Cooking time:*** *0 |* ***Servings:*** *2*

**Ingredients:**

- 6 tablespoons peanut butter
- 1/8 teaspoon salt
- 2 cups of milk

- 2 bananas
- 1/3 cup rolled oats
- 1 tablespoon protein powder

- 1 teaspoon honey
- 6-8 ice cubes

**Directions:**

Add oats in a blender and blend them well until it turns to a powder. Now peel the bananas and slice them. Add the sliced bananas in the blender with all the remaining ingredients. Blend all the ingredients together until combined. Add ice cubes in it and blend it well to chill the smoothie and to reach the required consistency. Add more milk or ice cubes as needed until the smoothie reaches your desired consistency. Now pour it in the serving glass and enjoy.

**Nutritional Information:** Carbohydrates 39g, Calories 370, Protein 14g, Fats: 17g, Sugar 9g.

### 17. Quinoa fruit salad
***Preparation time:*** *5 minutes |* ***Cooking time:*** *0 |* ***Servings:*** *4*

**Ingredients:**

- 2 cups properly cooked quinoa
- 1 teaspoon chopped mint leaves
- 1 peeled and cubed mango
- 2 tablespoons of nuts
- 1 tablespoon sugar

- ½ cup blueberries
- 1 cup diced strawberries
- ½ cup blueberries
- ¼ cup apple cider vinegar
- ¼ cup olive oil

- 3 tablespoons lemon juice
- 1 lemon zest

**Directions:**

Take a bowl and add vinegar, oil, sugar, lemon juice, and zest in the bowl and mix all the ingredients well. Put this bowl to the side. Now take another bowl and add mango, quinoa, nuts, blueberries, and strawberries. Whisk all the ingredients thoroughly. Now pour the mixed vinegar matter in the quinoa mixture and stir all the ingredients thoroughly. Move it to the serving bowl and garnish it with mint leaves and serve immediately.

**Nutritional Information:** Carbohydrates 34g, Calories 308, Protein 4g, Fats: 18g, Sugar 15g.

### 18. Almonds & nuts with oats
*Preparation time*: 5 minutes | *Cooking time*: 1 minute | *Servings*: 3

**Ingredients:**

- 1 cup almonds
- 3 cups oats
- 1 cup walnuts
- 1 cup crushed flaxseed
- 2 cups of milk
- 1 cup dried blueberries
- 1 cup brown sugar
- 1 ½ tablespoons cinnamon
- ½ tablespoon salt

**Directions:**

In a blender, blend one cup of oats, brown sugar, salt, almonds, and cinnamon. Blend all these ingredients thoroughly. Transfer the blended ingredients into a bowl. Now, add the remaining ingredients in the bowl and prepare the mixture and mix it well. Now, store the mixture in a bowl with a lid. Before serving it, add ¾ cup milk in the ½ cup prepared mixture and microwave it in a bowl for around one minute. Add the milk at the time of serving. You can also use water or almond milk instead of milk.

**Nutritional Information:** Carbohydrates 53g, Calories 355, Protein 9g, Fats: 13g, Sugar 19g.

### 19. Quinoa & chia porridge
*Preparation time: 5 minutes I **Cooking time**: 20 minutes I Servings: 1*

**Ingredients:**

- ¼ cup quinoa
- ½ cup milk
- ¼ teaspoon ground cinnamon
- ½ cup of water
- 1 tablespoon chia seed

**Directions:**

Take a pan and add milk and water in it and place it over a medium-high flame. When it comes to a boil, add quinoa, cinnamon and chia seeds and mix well. Now, reduce the heat and cover the pan with the lid. Cook it over a medium-low flame for around 12 to 15 minutes. Stir it frequently and cook it until the liquid is fully absorbed. When the quinoa starts to appear, remove it from the stove and set it aside for around 5 to 10 minutes to cool it down. After 5 minutes, serve it and if you want, you can top it with fruits, nuts, or milk.

**Nutritional Information:** Carbohydrates 51g, Calories 356, Protein 14g, Fats: 11g, Sugar 8g.

### 20. Peanut butter and banana pudding with chia seeds
*Preparation time: 5 minutes I **Chilling time**: 4 hours I Servings: 4*

**Ingredients:**

- 1 cup almond milk
- ½ cup peanut butter
- 1/2 cup yogurt
- 2 tablespoons honey

- ½ cup chia seeds
- 1 sliced banana
- 1 teaspoon vanilla extract
- 1 tablespoon roasted peanut

**Directions:**

Take a mixing bowl and combine the yogurt and butter and mix them well. Now, add vanilla extract, honey, chia seeds, and almond milk. Mix all the ingredients well until they become smooth. Pour the prepared mixture in a container and refrigerate it for at least 4 hours. After four hours, scoop the pudding in the serving bowl and garnish it with the banana slices and roasted peanuts. Now it is ready to serve.

**Nutritional Information:** Carbohydrates 34g, Calories 403, Protein 14g, Fats: 25g, Sugar 18g.

### 21. Banana zucchini oatmeal cups
**Preparation time**: 15 minutes I **Cooking time**: 25 minutes I **Servings**: 15

**Ingredients:**

- 2 cups grated zucchini
- 3 small mashed bananas
- ½ cup almond milk
- 1 teaspoon vanilla extract
- 1 tablespoon baking powder
- 3 tablespoons water
- ¼ cup maple syrup
- 3 cups oats
- 1 tablespoon crushed flaxseed
- 1 teaspoon cinnamon
- ¼ teaspoon salt

**Directions:**

Prepare the muffin tins with a muffin liner. Set the temperature of the oven to 375F. In a small bowl, mix flax and water and set it aside. In another bowl, combine the mashed bananas, almond milk, zucchini, maple syrup, and the prepared flax mixture. Stir all the ingredients well.

Add the remaining ingredients in it and mix it thoroughly. Now, pour the prepared mixture in the muffin tins and bake it in the preheated oven for around 23 to 25 minutes.

**Nutritional Information:** Carbohydrates 26g, Calories 215, Protein 5g, Fats: 3g, Sugar 9g.

22. Slow cooker sausages & egg casserole
    *Preparation time: 30 minutes I **Cooking time**: 06-08 hours I **Servings**: 10*

**Ingredients:**

- 12 eggs
- 16 ounces cooked and crumbled sausages
- ½ teaspoon black pepper
- ¼ cup milk
- 12 ounces grated cheddar cheese
- ¼ teaspoon garlic powder
- 32 ounces grated frozen hash browns
- 1 teaspoon salt
- 6 chopped onions

**Directions:**

Take a 6-quart slow cooker, and with the cooking spray, grease its insert. Now place the first layer of half hash browns in the cooker and sprinkle the salt and pepper. Now place the second layer of half sausages, then half onions and grated cheese. Repeat the layers in the same sequence and finish it by topping with cheese. Take a mixing bowl and mix eggs, salt, pepper, garlic powder, and milk. Whisk it well and pour it over the top layer. Cook for around 4 to 6 hours in the slow cooker over low heat.

**Nutritional Information:** Carbohydrates 17g, Calories 431, Protein 24g, Fats: 29g.

### 23. Cauliflower chaffle

*Preparation time: 5 minutes | Cooking time: 5 minutes | Servings: 2*

**Ingredients:**

- 1 egg
- ½ cup grated parmesan cheese
- ¼ teaspoon crushed black pepper
- ¼ teaspoon salt
- 1 cup rice cauliflower
- ½ cup grated mozzarella cheese
- ¼ teaspoon garlic powder
- ½ teaspoon Italian seasoning

**Directions:**

Mix all the ingredients, reserving 1/8 cup of parmesan cheese, into a blender and blend well. Now take a waffle maker and sprinkle the grated remaining parmesan cheese in it. Cover the waffle bottom with the cheese properly. Now fill the waffle maker with the prepared blended mixture. Now cover its top with the remaining cheese properly. Cook it for approximately 4 to 5 minutes or cook it until it becomes crispy and its color changes to a golden color. Make 4 mini chaffles with this batter and serve immediately.

**Nutritional Information:** Carbohydrates 7g, Calories 246, Protein 20g, Fats: 16g, Sugar 2g.

### 24. Garlic parmesan chaffle

*Preparation time: 5 minutes | Cooking time: 15 minutes | Servings: 2*

**Ingredients:**

- 1 egg
- ¾ teaspoon coconut flour
- 1 tablespoon parmesan
- 1/8 teaspoon Italian seasoning
- ¼ teaspoon garlic powder
- 1 tablespoon melted

cheese
- ¼ teaspoon basil seasoning
- A pinch of salt

butter
- 1 cup grated mozzarella cheese
- ¼ teaspoon baking powder

## Directions:

Preheat the oven to 400F temperature. Let the waffle maker get hot and grease it. Take a bowl and add eggs, half the mozzarella cheese, Parmesan cheese, flour, baking powder, Italian seasoning, and salt in it and stir all the ingredients well. Now scoop half of the prepared batter on the waffle maker and close it. Cook it for about 4 minutes. When it is cooked, remove it from the waffle and place it on a plate. In a bowl, mix the melted butter and garlic powder. Cut the cooked muffins into two pieces and brush the prepared garlic butter on its top. Place them in a baking pan and top it with the remaining mozzarella cheese. Bake it in the preheated oven for around 4 to 5 minutes. Remove it from the oven and before serving, sprinkle basil on top.

**Nutritional Information:** Carbohydrates 3g, Calories 270, Protein 16g, Fats: 21g, Sugar 1g.

### 25. Jalapeno & bacon chaffle
***Preparation time****: 5 minutes |* ***Cooking time****: 5 minutes |* ***Servings****: 5*

## Ingredients:

- 3 eggs
- 3 tablespoons coconut flour
- 3 washed, dried and de-seeded jalapeno peppers
- 1 teaspoon baking powder

- 4 slices bacon
- 8-ounces cream cheese
- ¼ teaspoon salt
- 1 cup grated cheese

**Directions:**

Take a pan and cook bacon over medium heat until it becomes crispy. In a bowl, mix salt, baking powder. and flour. In another bowl, beat cream cheese well. Preheat a greased waffle maker. Whisk eggs in another bowl and add half cream cheese and grated cheese. Add mixed dry ingredients and mix them well. In the end, mix jalapeno into the mixture. Scoop the batter into the waffle maker and cook it over medium heat for around 5 minutes. Transfer it to the serving plate and pour the remaining cream on it and serve.

**Nutritional Information:** Carbohydrates 5g, Calories 509, Protein 23g, Fats: 45g.

### 26. Chaffle garlic sticks
*Preparation time*: 3 minutes I *Cooking time*: 11 minutes I *Servings*: 2

**Ingredients:**

- 1 egg
- 1 cup grated Mozzarella cheese
- ½ teaspoon basil
- 1 tablespoon butter
- ½ teaspoon garlic powder
- 1 tablespoon almond flour

**Directions:**

Preheat the waffle maker. Take a mixing bowl combine egg, ¼ teaspoon garlic powder, ½ teaspoon basil, flour, and half cup Mozzarella cheese in it and mix it well. Add the half batter in the maker and cook for around 4 minutes. Cook the rest of the batter in the same way. Take another bowl and mix butter, remaining garlic powder. Microwave it for around 30 seconds. Now take a baking sheet and place the waffles on it. With the help of a brush spread the garlic butter on the waffle. Sprinkle cheese on the waffles and bake it for around 1 or 2 minutes at the 400 degrees' temperature or until the cheese melted.

**Nutritional Information:** Carbohydrates 2g, Calories 231, Protein 13g, Fats: 19g, Sugar 1g.

### 27. Avocado cucumber smoothie
***Preparation time**: 5 minutes I **Cooking time**: 0 I **Servings**: 1*

**Ingredients:**

- 1 avocado
- 1 cup almond milk
- 1 apple
- ½ tablespoon ground dill
- 1 teaspoon lemon juice
- ½ cucumber
- ¼ cup stalk celery

**Directions:**

Take the avocado and remove its stone. Dice and cut the celery and cucumber. Cut the apple into small cubes. Take a blender and put all the ingredients in it. Blend all the ingredients well until combined. If the consistency of smoothie is thicker, add more milk to it. When you reach your preferred consistency, transfer it to the serving glass. If you want the cold smoothie, then add ice cubes in it while blending.

**Nutritional Information:** Carbohydrates 21g, Calories 339, Protein 5g, Fats: 17g, Sugar 3g.

### 28. Sweet potato spinach bowl
***Preparation time**: 10 minutes I **Cooking time**: 15 minutes I Servings: 01*

**Ingredients:**

- ½ peeled, diced, sweet potatoes
- ¼ cup chopped fresh spinach
- ¼ cup ground walnuts
- ¼ cup vinegar
- ½ diced avocado
- ½ cup quinoa
- ¼ cup olive oil
- 3 teaspoons Dijon mustard

**Directions:**

For the dressing, in a mixing bowl, add oil, Dijon mustard, and vinegar.

Mix all these ingredients well and set it aside. Cook the quinoa according to the instructions given on the pack. Now take another medium-sized mixing bowl. Add quinoa, spinach, walnuts, sweet potato, and avocado in this mixing bowl. Mix all the ingredients properly. Now pour the prepared dressing on it and it is ready to serve.

**Nutritional Information:** Carbohydrates 42g, Calories 285, Protein 9g, Fats: 11g.

### 29. Mexican bean & avocado toast
**Preparation time**: 20 minutes I **Cooking time**: 10 minutes I **Servings**: 4

**Ingredients:**

- 1 ½ cup diced tomatoes
- 2 minced garlic cloves
- 1 sliced avocado
- 2 cans drained black beans
- 1 chopped onion
- 4 slices of bread
- 4 tablespoons olive oil
- 1 teaspoon lemon juice
- 1 teaspoon ground cumin
- 1 chopped bunch coriander
- 1 teaspoon chili flakes

**Directions:**

In a bowl, add ¼ onion, oil, and lemon juice. Mix these ingredients well. Place a skillet over a medium flame and fry the remaining onion in the oil. Add garlic and cook for an additional 1 minute. Now add chili flakes and cumin and cook for a few seconds. Now add beans and ¼ cup water, whisk it well and cook it. Add tomato and cook for an additional 1 minute. Season the cooked material with the coriander. Now, with the remaining oil, toast the bread. Place the toast on a serving plate and top it with the cooked batter. Serve it immediately.

**Nutritional Information:** Carbohydrates 30g, Calories 368, Protein 12g, Fats: 19g, Sugar 6g.

# Chapter 5: Recipes for Lunch

### 1. Vegan green bean casserole

*Preparation time*: 10 minutes | *Cooking time*: 20 minutes | *Servings*: 4

## Ingredients

- Green beans – 1 pound, cut in half
- Sea salt – to taste
- Shallot – 1, medium, minced
- Garlic – 2 cloves, minces
- Mushrooms – 1 cup, chopped
- Flour – 2 tablespoons
- Black pepper – to taste
- Butter – 2 tablespoons
- Vegetable broth – ¾ cup
- Almond milk (unsweetened) – 1 cup
- Fried onion – 1 ½ cup, divided

## Directions

Preheat the oven to 204 C or 400F. Take a large pot and bring water to boil. Add salt while water is boiling. Add green beans to the boiling water, allow it to boil for at least 5 minutes; drain and wash with cold water. Then drain the green beans properly and set them aside. Take a skillet, preferably oven-safe, heat the butter in it and put garlic and shallot. When the shallot starts to become translucent, add salt and pepper, and stir continuously. When the shallot is completely translucent, add finely chopped mushrooms to skillet and cook for another 4 to 5 minutes until the mushrooms become brown and cooked. Now add flour to the skillet and stir so it can combine well. Add vegetable broth slowly and whisk so the flour does not form any lumps in the liquid. Add almond milk and let it simmer. When it starts to simmer, reduce the heat to low and allow it to reduce until it reaches your desired thickness, or for about 7 minutes. When you reach the desired consistency, remove the skillet from heat and add 1/3 of fried onions and green beans. Toss until well combined. Sprinkle the rest of the fried onions on top. Bake the skillet for at least 15 minutes and heat in the oven until the top turns brown. Serve instantly!

## 2. Roasted vegetables

*Preparation time*: 15 minutes I *Cooking time*: 40 minutes I
*Servings*: 2

### Ingredients

- Butternut squash – 1, small, cubed
- Sweet potato – 1, cubed
- Yukon gold potatoes – 3, cubed
- Olive oil – ¼ cup
- Balsamic vinegar – 2 tablespoons
- Salt – to taste
- Red Bell pepper – 2, diced
- Red onion – 1, quartered
- Fresh thyme – 1 tablespoon
- Fresh rosemary – 2 tablespoons
- Black pepper – to taste

### Directions

Preheat the oven at 245C or 475F. Take a large bowl and add red bell pepper, butternut squash, sweet potatoes, red onion and Yukon gold potatoes. Take a small bowl and combine rosemary, thyme, balsamic vinegar, olive oil, black pepper, and salt. Add this mixture to the large bowl of vegetables; toss well so the mixture can combine with the vegetables evenly. Take a roasting pan, brush with oil, and spread the vegetables on it evenly. Put the pan into the preheated oven and roast for at least 40 minutes or until the vegetables are properly cooked. Stir after every 10 minutes. Serve warm!

### 3. Cauliflower stuffing

*Preparation time*: 15 minutes | *Cooking time*: 40 minutes | *Servings*: 6

## Ingredients

- Onion – 1, chopped
- Celery stalks – 2, chopped
- Cauliflower – 1 small, chopped
- Mushrooms – 1 cup, chopped
- Rosemary – 2 tablespoons, chopped
- Sage – 1 tablespoon, freshly chopped
- Butter – 4 tablespoons
- Carrot – 2, large, peeled, chopped
- Black pepper – grounded, to taste
- Parsley – ¼ cup, chopped
- Chicken broth – ½ cup

## Directions

Take a large pan or skillet, melt the butter over medium heat, add celery, onion and carrot, and cook for 8 minutes until soft. Add mushrooms and cauliflower and freshly grounded black pepper and salt, then cook for 10 minutes until tender. Now add rosemary, parsley and sage and stir well. Add chicken broth to the skillet and cook for 10 minutes until the liquid is absorbed by the vegetables. Serve warm!

### 4. Chicken lettuce wraps

*Preparation time*: 30 minutes | *Cooking time*: 20 minutes | *Servings*: 4

## Ingredients

- Hoisin sauce – 5 tablespoons
- Soy sauce – 2 tablespoons
- Rice vinegar – 2 tablespoons
- Sesame oil – 1 teaspoon
- Turkey – 1 pound
- Garlic – 3 cloves, minced
- Cornstarch – 1 teaspoon
- Vegetable oil – 2 teaspoons, divided
- Mushrooms – 8 ounces, chopped
- Onion, carrots, bell pepper –

- Ginger – 1 tablespoon, freshly minced
- Scallions – ½ cup, thin sliced, divided
- diced (Optional)
- Chestnuts – 1 can, finely chopped
- Butter lettuce – 2 heads, small
- Hot sauce, red pepper flakes – for garnish

**Directions**

Take a small bowl, combine hoisin sauce, rice vinegar, soy sauce and sesame oil. For a thicker sauce, you can add cornstarch. Take a large pan or skillet, heat the oil at a medium temperature, put the turkey into the pan and cook for 8 to 10 minutes until cooked and the pink color of the meat vanishes; set aside. In the same pan, heat the oil, add the vegetables (optional ones) and mushrooms, and stir and cook for 5 minutes until tender. Stir in ginger, chestnuts and garlic; cook for about a minute until fragrant. Add the cooked turkey into the pan and add half of the scallions; combine well. Now add the sauce into the pan and cook for another minute until it bubbles. Separate the leaves of lettuce from its branch and pile them. Put the chicken material into each leaf. Garnish with scallions, red pepper flakes and hot sauce according to your taste.

5. **Zucchini sushi**
   *Preparation time: 20 minutes | **Cooking time**: 20 minutes | **Servings**: 2*

**Ingredients**

- Zucchini – 2, medium
- Crab meat – 1 can
- Carrot – ½ thinly cut
- Avocado – ½ unit, diced
- Cucumber – ½ unit, thinly cut
- Cream cheese – 4 oz.
- Hot sauce – 1 teaspoon
- Lime juice – 1 teaspoon
- Sesame seeds – 1 tablespoon, toasted

## Directions

With the help of a vegetable peeler, thinly slice the zucchini in flat strips; put the stripes on a paper towel to sit. Take a medium bowl, whisk hot sauce, cream cheese and lime juice; set aside. Take 2 strips of zucchini, spread the cream cheese mixture on top, add pinch of avocado, crab, carrot and cucumber and roll it. Repeat with the rest of the strips. Sprinkle sesame seeds on top before serving.

### 6. Avocado, beans and chicken salad
*Preparation time*: 13 minutes I *Cooking time*: 7 minutes I *Servings*: 4

## Ingredients

- Olive oil – 3 tablespoons
- Chili powder – 1 tablespoon
- Garlic – 4 cloves, minced
- Black beans – 1 can, rinsed
- Salt – to taste
- Green onion – 2 units, sliced
- Avocado – 2, diced
- Cilantro – 1/3 cup
- Cayenne pepper – 1 pinch
- Boneless chicken breast – 1.25 pound – diced
- Cumin 1 tablespoon
- Black pepper – to taste
- Cherry tomatoes – 2 cups, halved
- Lime juice – 4 tablespoons
- Apple cider vinegar – 2 tablespoons
- Honey – 3 tablespoons

## Directions

Take a large skillet and heat olive oil at medium heat. Add chicken, chili powder, and cumin. Cook for about 5 minutes until done. Add garlic and cook for another minute until fragrant. Add the beans, black pepper, and salt. Stir well until combined. Transfer the mixture into a large bowl. Add green onions, tomatoes, avocado, apple cider vinegar, cilantro and lime juice; stir and combine. Add the cayenne, honey and remaining salt and pepper;. Your meal is ready to be served.

### 7. Avocado stuffed shrimp salad

*Preparation time*: 10 minutes I *Cooking time*: 15 minutes I *Servings*: 4

## Ingredients

- Cooked Shrimps – ½ pound, chopped
- Celery – ½ cup
- Parsley – 1 tablespoon
- Dijon Mustard – 2 teaspoons
- Lemon juice – 1 ½ teaspoons
- Tarragon – ¾ teaspoon, dried
- Onion – ¼ cup, chopped
- Mayonnaise – 3 tablespoons
- Capers – 4 teaspoons, drained
- Seasoned salt – ¼ teaspoon
- Pepper – 1/8 teaspoon
- Avocado – 2 medium unit, halved

### Directions

In a bowl, combine shrimp, onion, celery, mayonnaise, parsley, capers, Dijon mustard, salt, pepper, lemon juice and tarragon. Take the avocado and fill this mixture in the center. Serve immediately!

### 8. Fajita steak salad bowl

*Preparation time*: 10 minutes I *Cooking time*: 15 minutes I *Servings*: 4

## Ingredients

- Lettuce – 7 ounces
- Steak of your choice – 1 lb.
- Olive oil – 4 tablespoons, divided
- Bell pepper – 2 cups, strips
- Corn tortillas – 2
- Mexican crema sauce – ½ cup
- Lime juice – 2 tablespoons
- Chili powder – 2 tablespoons
- Cumin – 1 teaspoon, grounded
- Smoked paprika – 1 teaspoon
- Onion powder – 1 teaspoon
- Red onion – ½, sliced
- Corn – 1
- Black olives – ¼ cup
- Cherry tomatoes – 4, halved
- Fresh cilantro – ½ cup
- Fajita seasoning – ½ tablespoon
- Salt – 1 teaspoon, divided
- Sugar – 1 teaspoon
- Oregano – ½ teaspoon
- Cayenne pepper – ½ teaspoon
- Black pepper – ½ teaspoon

- Garlic powder – 1 teaspoon
- Cilantro & jalapenos – for garnish

**Directions**

Take tortilla and cut it in half. Then cut it into strips almost about ¼ inch of width. Take a large skillet and heat the olive oil on high heat. Add the strips and fry for few minutes, flip and cook until golden brown; drain the oil and dry with paper towel. Season with salt.

In a blender, add chili powder, cumin, paprika, onion powder, garlic powder, sugar, oregano, cayenne pepper, salt and black pepper; blend to combine. Now your fajita seasoning is ready.

Take food processor, add Mexican Crema Sauce, lime juice, cilantro, previously prepared fajita seasoning, and a pinch of salt; process to make a smooth dressing for the salad. Pat dry the steak and apply a generous amount of fajita seasoning on both sides. Take the same skillet and heat the oil on high flame; put steak in the hot oil and cook for 3 minutes from each side; remove from the skillet and let the steak rest for at least 10 minutes. Wipe the remains from the skillet and heat another tablespoon of olive oil; put onion, sear for a minute at high flame, remove from pan. Repeat this process with the peppers. Take the corn cob and flame it over on the flame to get the kernels until charred and popped. Layer the lettuce in a large salad bowl; slice the prepared steak into strips and arrange it with salad, olives, pepper and onions, corm, tortilla strips and the rest. Top your salad with the dressing Garnish with jalapenos and cilantro.

9. **Grilled chicken with asparagus & white beans**
   *Preparation time*: 10 minutes I *Cooking time*: 15 minutes I
   *Servings*: 4

**Ingredients**

- Chicken breast - 4
- Asparagus – 12 stalks
- Garlic – 2 cloves
- Parsley – ½ cup

- Oil – 1 tablespoon
- Cannellini beans – 800 g
- Salt & pepper – 1 teaspoon
- Olive oil – ½ cup
- Lemon juice – ¼ cup
- Dijon mustard – 1 teaspoon

### Directions

Apply olive oil on both sides of the chicken and sprinkle salt over it. Take a frying pan and heat the heat a tablespoon of oil; cook chicken in it for 5 minutes from each side until tender. In a pot, boil water with a pinch of water; add asparagus and let it boil until tender; drain. In a small bowl, combine cannellini beans with garlic, onion and parsley. Now add lemon juice, oil, Dijon mustard, pepper and salt in the bean bowl and combine. Slice the chicken; serve with the white bean salad and boiled asparagus.

### 10. Cardamom chicken with lime leaves
*Preparation time*: 30 minutes I *Cooking time*: 1 Hour 15 minutes I *Servings*: 4

### Ingredients

- Rapeseed – 2 tablespoons
- Onion – 1, chopped
- Ginger – 2 tablespoons, grated
- Garlic – 4 cloves, grated
- Cardamom pods – 12, lightly crushed
- Red chili – 1, halved
- Tomatoes – 400g, chopped
- Mango chutney – 1 tablespoon
- Vegetable bouillon powder – 3 teaspoons, divided
- Basmati rice – 125g
- Red lentils – 100g
- Cloves – 4
- Cinnamon stick – 1
- Turmeric – 3 teaspoons, halved
- White pepper – 1 ½ teaspoons
- Coriander – 1 teaspoon, grounded
- Cumin – 1 teaspoon
- Auvergne – 1, cubed
- Lime leaves – 4
- Boneless chicken – 1kg
- Green pepper – 1, sliced
- Cumin seeds – 1 teaspoon

## Directions

Take a large pan and heat the oil; add onion and cook it for 5 minutes until translucent. Put garlic, cardamom, ginger, cinnamon and cloves in the pan; cook for another 5 minutes. Add the rest of the spices into the pan, tomatoes, mango chutney, water and bouillon. Now add Auvergne into the pan; boil the mixture, then let it simmer for at least 15 minutes. Add lime leaves and chicken into the pan, cover it and allow it to cook for at least 40 minutes. After the chicken is cooked, remove the chicken from the pan, shred it into medium pieces, and return it to the pan again. In a saucepan, add 750ml of water, boil the rice along with red lentils, cumin seeds, turmeric and bouillon powder; cover and allow it to cook for at least 20 minutes until rice is tender. Turn off the heat and leave it until the moisture absorbs. Serve the rice with the chicken curry!

### 11. Chicken Caesar wraps
*Preparation time*: 15 minutes I *Cooking time*: 0 minutes I *Servings*: 6

## Ingredients

- Caesar salad dressing – ¾ cup
- Parmesan cheese – ¼ cup, grated
- Garlic powder – ½ teaspoon
- Cooked chicken breast – 3 cups
- Torn romaine – 2 cups
- Caesar salad croutons – ¾ cup, chopped
- Whole wheat tortillas – 6

## Directions

Take a large bowl. Combine dressing, garlic powder, cheese and pepper. Add romaine, chicken and croutons. Take a tortilla, spread over 2/3 cup of the mixture and roll it up. Serve fresh!

### 12. Sweet potato with broccoli & white beans
*Preparation time*: 15 minutes I *Cooking time*: 15 minutes I *Servings*: 4

**Ingredients**

- Organic broccoli – 8 cups, chopped
- Garlic – 3 cloves, minced
- Sweet potato – 1 medium
- Vegetable broth – 2 cups
- Paprika – ½ teaspoon
- Yeast – 1/3 cup
- White beans – 1 ½ cup
- Onion – 1, chopped
- Black pepper – ¾ teaspoon
- Salt – ¼ teaspoon
- Bay leaf – 1 leaf
- Cooked pasta 1 cup (optional)

**Directions**

In a large pot, bring the water to boil. Add sweet potato and let it boil for 6 minutes until tender. Add broccoli and let it boil for another 3 minutes. After exactly 10 minutes, drain the water away. Place 2/3 of the broccoli in a blender and set aside the rest. Add ½ the sweet potatoes in the blender and set aside the rest. Add half chopped onion into the blender; add yeast, beans, salt, pepper, broth, paprika and garlic. Blend the ingredients well until you get a thick and smooth consistency. Pour this mixture into a pot. Add the rest of the vegetables and bay leaf; boil the mixture and reduce the heat and let it simmer for 5 minutes. If you are using pasta, than do not cook it for long the mixture as it will get mushy. Serve the soup hot!

### 13. Salmon pasta with lemon
*Preparation time*: 5 minutes I *Cooking time*: 20 minutes I *Servings*: 4

**Ingredients**

- Salmon – 1 pound, boneless
- Garlic – 2 cloves, sliced
- Unsalted butter – 4 tablespoons
- Olive oil – 1 tablespoon
- Lemon wedges – for garnish
- Lemon juice – 3 tablespoons
- Salt – to taste
- Black Pepper – to taste
- Pasta of your choice – ½ lb.
- Parsley – ¼ cup

## Directions

Preheat the oven to 199C or 390F. Pat dry the salmon with a paper towel and place it on a baking dish. Apply black pepper and salt all over the fillet; top with garlic slices, olive oil and lemon juice. Bake the fillet for about 15 minutes until done. Take out the dish from the oven and allow it to cool; flake out the fillet into a bit larger pieces (it will break while tossing). Take a medium pan and cook pasta along with parsley; you can also add dill if you like. When the pasta is done, drain it and add salmon chunks along with the juice; toss well to combine. Add more lemon juice if desired. Season with black pepper, salt and lemon wedges. Serve readily!

### 14. Roasted tomato soup

*Preparation time*: 20 minutes I *Cooking time*: 50 minutes I *Servings*: 4-6

## Ingredients

- Tomatoes - 2 ½ pound
- Garlic – 5 cloves, peeled
- Yellow onion – 2, sliced
- Olive oil – ½ cup
- Heavy cream – ¾ cup (Optional)
- Basil leaves – ½ cup, chopped (Optional)
- Black pepper – to taste
- Salt – to taste
- Chick stock – 1 quart
- Bay leaves – 2
- Butter – 4 tablespoons
- Vine cherry tomato – for garnish (optional)

## Directions

Preheat the oven at 232C or 450F. Cut the tomatoes in half and put them on a baking tray along with onion slices and garlic clove; if you are using tomatoes for garnishing, then put them to the side as well. Shower the extra virgin olive oil, black pepper and salt all over the tomatoes. Put the tray in the oven and allow it to bake for at least 30 minutes until the tomatoes are caramelized. Separate the tomatoes you put for the garnish and transfer the rest of the material into a pot. Add chicken stock, remaining butter and bay leaves into the pot; cook until starts boil, simmer for at least 20 minutes until reduced to a third at low heat. Add basil leaves (if using); remove bay leaves and add the remaining puree into the blender to make a smooth soup texture. Again, transfer the soup into the pot and heat at low flame; add heavy cream (if using) and get your required consistency (use more chicken stock if required). Serve with the roasted tomatoes, grounded black pepper, salt and a splash of heavy cream on top.

### 15. Green peas and lentil soup

*Preparation time*: 10 minutes | *Cooking time*: 40 minutes | *Servings*: 4

## Ingredients

- Green lentils – 350 grams
- Green peas – 350 grams
- Shallot – 120 grams
- Carrots – 3 oz.
- Garlic – 1 clove
- Salt – to taste
- Cheese – 4 tablespoons
- Vegetable broth – 2 liters
- Olive oil – 10 tablespoons
- Parsley – 1 bunch
- Black peppercorn – to taste

## Directions

Soak the lentils in water for at least 10 minutes. Take a pan or a pot, heat 3 tablespoons of olive oil and stir fry shallot, garlic and carrots. When the shallot turns translucent, add the green peas and lentils; cook for 5 minutes than add vegetable broth and bring to boil. Once the broth gets to boiling point, reduce the heat, cover the pot and let it simmer until get soup for at least 40 minutes or so. When the soup is ready add black peppercorn and salt to taste. Serve with the topping of parsley, Parmigiano Reggiano Cheese (or cheese of your choice) with olive oil. Serve hot!

### 16. Grilled chicken salad sandwich

*Preparation time*: 15 minutes | *Cooking time*: 15 minutes | *Servings*: 4

## Ingredients

- Mayonnaise – 1 cup
- Black pepper – 1/8 teaspoon
- Garlic powder – 1/8 teaspoon
- Celery salt – 1/8 teaspoon
- Grilled chicken – 4 cups
- Tomato – 1, sliced
- Celery stalks – 2, sliced
- Dried cranberries – ½ cup
- Cashews – 2/3 cup
- Bread slice – 8, toasted
- Lettuce – 4 leaves

## Directions

In a bowl, combine mayonnaise, garlic powder, black pepper and celery salt. Add cranberries, chicken, celery and cashews in the same bowl and combine until a mixture formed. Apply the mayonnaise mixture on the toasted bread slice; place lettuce and tomato slice; sandwich with the other bread slice.

### 17. Vegetable barley soup

*Preparation time*: 5 minutes | *Cooking time*: 50 minutes | *Servings*: 6

## Ingredients

- Yellow onion – 1
- Garlic – 2 cloves
- Olive oil – 2 tablespoons
- Carrot – 4
- Tomato – 1 can, diced
- Barley – 1 cup
- Peas – ½ cup
- Lemon juice – 1 tablespoon
- Basil – ½ teaspoon, dried
- Oregano – ½ teaspoon, dried
- Black pepper – to taste
- Vegetable broth – 6 cups
- Russet potato – 1
- Green beans = 1 cup
- Corn – ½ cup
- Parsley – 1 handful, for garnish

## Directions

In a pot, heat olive oil; dice garlic and onion on medium heat for around 5 minutes until translucent. Add carrots, tomatoes, basil, barley, oregano, vegetable broth and black pepper; cook for few minutes until the mixture starts to boil; reduce the heat to medium low and let the soup simmer for at least 30 minutes; stir occasionally. Meanwhile, peel and dice the potato into cubes. Check for the barley if it's cooked, then add potatoes into the pot and let it cook for another 10 minutes until tender. Add corn, green beans and peas into the pot; cook for another 5 minutes until well combined. In the end, add lemon juice, adjust the pepper and salt according to your taste. Serve hot with parsley garnished on top!

### 18. Parmesan Brussels sprouts
*Preparation time*: 10 minutes | *Cooking time*: 45 minutes | *Servings*: 4

## Ingredients

- Brussels sprouts – 12 ounces, halved
- Olive oil – 2 tablespoons
- Salt – to taste
- Black pepper – to taste
- Parmesan – 1 cup, shredded
- Cooking spray

## Directions

Preheat the oven at 218C or 425F; place a cast-iron skillet in the oven as well. In a medium bowl, toss Brussels sprouts with salt, olive oil and black pepper; add parmesan in the end. Remove the skillet from the oven carefully, spray the cooking oil generously. Spread the Brussels sprouts in the skillet; put back the skillet into the oven and aloe it to bake for about 25 minutes until the Brussels sprouts are brown and tender. Serve warm!

### 19. Chicken steak soup

*Preparation time:* 5 minutes I *Cooking time:* 40 minutes I *Servings:* 6

## Ingredients

- Butter – 2 tablespoons
- Vegetable oil – 2 tablespoons
- Chicken steak – 1 ½ pound
- Onion – ½ cup, chopped
- All-purpose flour – 3 tablespoons
- Paprika – 1 tablespoon
- Celery – 1 ½ cup, chopped
- Tomato paste – 1 can
- Corn – 1 can, drained
- Carrot – 1 ½ cup, sliced
- Salt – 1 teaspoon
- Black pepper – ¼ teaspoon, grounded
- Chicken broth – 4 cups
- Water 1 cup
- Parsley – ½ cup, chopped
- Celery leaves – 3 tablespoons, chopped
- Bay leaf – 1
- Marjoram – ½ teaspoon, dried
- Yukon gold potato – 1 ½ cup, diced

## Directions

Take a skillet and melt the butter on medium heat; stir the steak pieces in the butter along with onions. Cook for 10 minutes until browned. Meanwhile, in a small bowl, combine flour, salt, paprika and black pepper; sprinkle it over the chicken steak pieces and coat well. Take a large pot for soup, add broth, parsley, water, celery leaves, marjoram and bay leaf; add the steak mixture as well; boil the mixture and stir in intervals. When the mixture starts to boil, reduce the flame and let it simmer for about 30 minutes until tender. Add carrots, potato, celery, tomato paste and the corn in the soup let it simmer for another 15 minutes until tender. Remove the bay leaf before serving

### 20. Lemon garlic shrimp
***Preparation time****: 5 minutes | **Cooking time***: *15 minutes |*
***Servings****: 4*

## Ingredients

- Butter – 2 tablespoons, divided
- Olive oil – 1 tablespoon
- Shrimp – 1 lb., deveined
- Lemon – 1, sliced
- Lemon juice – 1 tablespoon
- Garlic – 3 cloves, minced
- Red pepper flakes – 1 teaspoon, crushed
- Kosher salt – to taste
- Dry white wine – 2 tablespoons
- Parsley – ½ cup, chopped, for garnish

## Directions

Take a large skillet and melt butter and olive oil over medium heat; stir shrimp for a minute; add garlic, lemon slices and red pepper flakes along with salt. Cook for about 3 minutes per side until shrimp tenders. Once the shrimp turns pink, remove the skillet from heat; add remaining butter, white wine and lemon juice. Garnish with chopped parsley and sprinkle some salt before serving.

### 21. Shrimp cucumber bites
***Preparation time****: 20 minutes | **Cooking time***: *30 minutes |*
***Servings****: 6*

## Ingredients

- Olive oil – 1/3 cup
- Lime juice – 4 tablespoons, divided
- Honey – 2 tablespoons
- Garlic – 2 cloves, minced
- Cilantro – 2 tablespoons, for garnish
- Cucumber – 2, thick sliced
- Cajun seasoning – 1 teaspoon
- Kosher salt – to taste
- Shrimp – 1 lb., deveined
- Avocados – 2
- Red onion – ½ minced
- Jalapeno – 1, chopped

## Directions

Take a large bowl, combine lime juice, olive oil, honey, Cajun seasoning, salt and garlic. Add shrimp in the bowl, coat well and refrigerate for about 30 minutes or more. Take a large skillet. On a medium heat cook the shrimp until tender. It will not take more than 2 minutes or so. Remove the skillet from the heat. Take another bowl and mash avocados, add red onion, lime juice, cilantro, salt and jalapeno. Take a cucumber slice, spread the avocado spread (guacamole) over each slice; place shrimp on top and garnish with cilantro.

### 22. Balsamic glazed shrimp with quinoa
*Preparation time: 15 minutes | Cooking time: 25 minutes | Servings: 4*

## Ingredients

- Quinoa – 1 cup
- Parsley – 1 cup, divided
- Shrimp – 1 lb., deveined
- Olive oil – 3 tablespoons, divided
- Kosher salt – to taste
- Dry white wine – ½ cup
- Sugar – 2 tablespoons
- Black pepper – to taste
- Garlic – 2 cloves, minced
- Orange juice – 2 cups
- Orange zest – 1 tablespoon
- Lemon juice – 1 tablespoon
- Balsamic vinegar – 2 tablespoons

## Directions

Preheat the oven to 400F. Take a medium pot and prepare quinoa by following the directions given on the box. Sprinkle parsley over the cooked quinoa and set it aside. Pat dry the shrimp, put olive oil, black pepper and salt over them evenly. Take a baking tray, place the shrimp evenly and bake them for about 9 minutes until turned pink. Take a large skillet, heat the olive oil on medium low flame. Add garlic, black pepper, salt, orange zest, balsamic vinegar, lemon juice, orange juice, white wine and sugar. Increase the flame and cook until it boils; when it starts to boil, lower the heat a bit and let the sauce simmer for about 10 minutes until reduced. Take out the shrimp from the oven and toss it in the balsamic sauce. Serve with quinoa and garnish with parsley.

### 23. Vegetarian chickpea sandwich
*Preparation time*: 20 minutes | *Cooking time*: 0 minutes | *Servings*: 4

## Ingredients

- Chickpeas – 1 can, rinsed
- Celery – 1 stalk, chopped
- Onion – ½, chopped
- Mayonnaise – 1 tablespoon
- Bread – 8 slices
- Lemon juice – 1 tablespoon
- Dill weed – 1 teaspoon, dried
- Salt – to taste
- Pepper – to taste

## Directions

Take a medium bowl, put drained and rinsed chickpeas in it and mash them with a help of a fork. Add lemon juice, celery, mayonnaise, onion, salt, dill and pepper; mix well to form a mixture. Spread this mixture on the bread slice and sandwich it with another slice.

### 24. California chicken avocado wrap
*Preparation time*: 15 minutes | *Cooking time*: 8 minutes | *Servings*: 4

## Ingredients

- Turkey bacon – 8 slices
- Chicken – 2 cups, shredded
- Salt – to taste
- Pepper – to taste
- Mango – 1, chopped
- Mayonnaise – 6 tablespoons, divided
- Lime juice – 2 tablespoons
- Avocado – 1 large
- Whole wheat tortillas – 4
- Romaine – 2 cups, shredded
- Tomato – 1, diced

## Directions

Take a large skillet and cook turkey bacon strips until crispy; set aside in paper towel plate. Take a large bowl, combine shredded chicken, black pepper, salt, mayonnaise, mango and lime juice. In another bowl, peel the avocado and mash; add the remaining mayonnaise, black pepper and salt; mix well and set aside. Take a tortilla, spread the avocado mixture over it leaving an inch boarder; put the lettuce, 2 turkey bacon slices and tomato. Spread the chicken mixture over the veggies; roll up the tortilla like a burrito. Cut each of the rolled-up tortilla in half before serving.

### 25. Baked eggs in avocado
*Preparation time*: 10 minutes | *Cooking time*: 15 minutes | *Servings*: 6

## Ingredients

- Avocado – 2, halved
- Egg – 6
- Black pepper and salt – to taste
- Chives – 2 tablespoons, freshly chopped

## Directions

Preheat the oven at 213C or 425F. Take a baking tray and coat it with generous amount of cooking spray. Scoop out some avocado from the mid of each halved unit to make space. Crack 1 egg gently inside the space of the avocado; season with black pepper and salt. Place the avocados in the oven and bake them for around 15 minutes until the egg white sets. Garnish with chives and serve immediately.

### 26. Skillet steak with corn salad
*Preparation time*: 10 minutes | *Cooking time*: 30 minutes | *Servings*: 4

## Ingredients

- Boneless beef steak – 1 pound,
- Beef broth – ¾ cup

strips
- Onion – 1, wedges
- Thyme – ½ teaspoon, dried
- Canola oil – 2 tablespoons

- Tomatoes – 1 can, diced
- Corn – 2 cans, drained
- Cooked rice – for serving

**Directions**

Take a large skillet, heat the oil, cook beefsteaks along with thyme and onion on medium heat for about 15 minutes until pinkish color disappears. Drain out the excess water; add wine and let it simmer for about 10 minutes until the liquid evaporates completely. Stir the diced tomatoes and again let it simmer for 15 minutes. Add the corn in the last and let it heat a bit. Serve with cooked rice!

### 27. Chicken stir fry
*Preparation time*: 30 minutes | *Cooking time*: 35 minutes | *Servings*: 6

**Ingredients**

- White rice – 2 cups
- Water – 4 cups
- Soy sauce – 2/3 cup
- Brown sugar – ¼ cup
- Cornstarch – 1 tablespoon
- Ginger – 1 tablespoon, freshly minced
- Garlic – 1 tablespoon, minced
- Red pepper flakes – ¼ teaspoon

- Chicken breast – 3, boneless, sliced
- Sesame oil – 2 tablespoons, divided
- Bell pepper – 1, sliced
- Water chestnuts – 2 can, sliced
- Broccoli – 1 head, broken
- Carrots – 1 cup, sliced
- Onion – 1, large chunks

## Directions

In a saucepan, boil water along with rice; reduce the heat to low, cover and allow to simmer until the water evaporates the from rice, for about 25 minutes. In a small bowl, combine brown sugar, soy sauce and corn starch; add garlic, ginger and red pepper and mix. Marinate the chicken with the sauce and refrigerate for at least 15 minutes. Take a skillet and heat the sesame oil over medium high heat; stir the water chestnuts, bell pepper, carrots, broccoli and onion until tender; remove these vegetables from skillet and set aside. Take out the chicken and save the marinate. Heat the sesame oil and cook chicken in the skillet on medium high heat until the pink color disappears, almost 3 minutes per side. When the chicken is half cooked, return the vegetables into the pan along with the reserved marinate material. Boil the material and cook for 7 minutes until the chicken is properly done. Serve with rice!

### 28. Pasta with broccoli and tomato sauce

*Preparation time*: 10 minutes | *Cooking time*: 20 minutes | *Servings*: 2

## Ingredients

- Pasta – 6 oz.
- Broccoli – ½ lb.
- Garlic – 2 cloves, chopped
- Shallot – 1, chopped
- Capers – 1 tablespoon
- Calabrian Chile pasta - 1 ½ teaspoon
- Parmesan cheese – ¼ cup, grated
- Tomato paste – 2 tablespoons
- Mascarpone cheese – 2 tablespoons

## Directions

In a pot, boil water with a pinch of salt. Meanwhile, cut the broccoli head into ½ inches. Put the pasta in the boiling water and cook for 5 minutes. After 5 minutes, put broccoli in the pot as well and allow it to boil until tender for around another 5 minutes. Reserve ½ cup of the boiling water and drain the rest. In a medium pan heat the olive oil on medium heat; add shallot, garlic and capers; stir for a minute until translucent; add Chile paste and tomato paste. Allow to cook for 2 minutes, stir continuously. Add the ½ cup of reserved water into the pan and cook for another 2 minutes until thickened. Add salt and black pepper to taste. Remove the sauce from heat. Add cooked broccoli, pasta and mascarpone. Combine and heat for another 2 minutes so the pasta can coat completely. Serve with garnished Parmesan cheese.

### 29. Salmon with lemon and dill

*Preparation time*: 10 minutes I *Cooking time*: 25 minutes I
*Servings*: 2

**Ingredients**

- Salmon – 1 pound
- Butter – ¼ cup
- Lemon juice – 5 tablespoons
- Dill weed – 1 tablespoon, dried
- Garlic powder – ¼ teaspoon
- Salt – to taste
- Black pepper – to taste

**Directions**

Preheat the oven to 175C or 350F. Grease the baking dish with oil. In a small bowl, combine butter and lemon juice; place the salmon fillets into the baking tray and drizzle over the butter mixture onto it; season garlic powder, dill, pepper and salt all over the fillet. Place the dish into the oven and bake for about 25 minutes until salmon is flaked with the help of fork. Serve hot!

### 30. Barbeque halibut steak

*Preparation time: 10 minutes I **Cooking time**: 15 minutes I*
*Servings: 2*

## Ingredients

- Halibut steak – 1 pound
- Butter – 2 tablespoons
- Brown sugar – 2 tablespoons
- Garlic – 2 cloves, minced
- Soy sauce – 2 teaspoons
- Black pepper – ½ teaspoon, grounded
- Lemon juice – 1 tablespoon

## Directions

Preheat the barbeque grill at medium high heat. In a small saucepan, add brown sugar, butter, garlic, soy sauce, lemon juice and pepper; heat the pan over medium heat until sugar dissolves; stir occasionally. Oil the grill, Brush the brown sugar sauce on to the halibut steak and place them on the grill; cook each side for about 5 minutes until done. Serve hot!

# Chapter 6: Recipes for Dinner

### 1. Mushroom and Veggie Soup

*Preparation time*: 20 minutes I *Cooking time*: 30 minutes I *Servings*: 5-6 persons

### Ingredients:

- 3 tbsp. Olive/vegetable oil
- 1 diced yellow onion
- Minced garlic cloves
- 1 diced zucchini
- 1 tsp dried thyme
- 3-4 bay leaves

- 8 cups vegetable sodium broth
- 12 ounces trimmed and chopped mushrooms
- 2 cups florets of broccoli
- 1/4 cup Soy sauce
- 1 tsp oregano
- Optional to enhance flavor- 1 tbsp apple cider vinegar

### Directions:

In a stockpot, add up oil and onion in it. Sauté the onion for a good amount of time, about 7 minutes, until it has turned soft while maintaining to stir recurrently. Now add garlic to the pot and sauté it till it turns aromatic. Add mushrooms, zucchini, thyme, bay leaves, vegetable broth, broccoli, soy sauce, and oregano and simmer the mixture until good lot of 15 minutes. Add salt and vinegar for appeasing and enhancing flavor, depending on your preference.

### 2. Potato and Almond Soup

*Preparation time*: 30 minutes I *Cooking time*: 30 minutes I *Servings*: 4-5 cups/ 2-4 persons

### Ingredients:

- 2 medium sized potato
- 4 garlic cloves
- 1 onion
- Kosher salt (sea salt)

- 2 tbsp. virgin olive oil
- 2 cups water
- 1 cup blanched almonds
- 2 tbsp. apple cider vinegar

- 2 thyme
- Grounded black pepper

**Directions:**

Set the oven to 450 degrees to preheat it, and line the baking tray with aluminum foil. Take peeled potatoes in a bowl and chop them into chunks. In a similar manner, peel onions and chop them to chunk size. Next, peel the garlic cloves and chop them coarsely. Place both the elements in the bowl alongside the potatoes and drizzle oil over the mixture before spreading in on the baking tray/sheet. Let the mixture be roasted for a good lot of 15 to 20 minutes so that it turns out to be tender. Bring almonds to simmer in a pot and let it be cooked for 2 straight minutes before combining it and the roasted batter in a blender. Add salt, thyme and black pepper over to brighten up the flavor as required.

3. **Red Lentil Salsa Soup**
   *Preparation time*: 10-15 minutes | *Cooking time*: 30-45 minutes | *Servings*: 9 cups/6 persons

**Ingredients:**

- 1 tbsp. Olive oil
- 2 medium sized diced onions
- 3 Diced carrots
- 3 Minced cloves of garlic
- 3 tsp Cumin
- 3 tsp Oregano dried
- Broth (vegetable or chicken - 4 cups)
- 3 cups water
- 1.5-2 cups green lentils, dried
- 2 cups salsa

**Directions:**

Heat oil in a stockpot and add onions and carrots to it. Stir the mixture for about 7 minutes, until it becomes tender. Sauté garlic, oregano, and cumin while repetitively whipping it for total of 30 seconds. Insert water, broth, salsa, and lentils into the heated pot and bring it to boil proceeded by simmering it until lentils become soft. Garnish thyme and parsley over the soup and to brighten up your taste. Voila! Bon appetite!

4. **Garlic pasta with roasted Brussels sprouts and tomatoes**
   *Preparation time*: 10 minutes I *Cooking time*: 35-40 minutes I
   *Servings*: 7-8 cups/4 persons

**Ingredients:**

- 15 Fairly sliced Brussels sprouts
- 30 grape or datterini tomatoes
- 1 garlic clove
- 1 tsp olive oil
- 11 oz spaghetti
- 5-6 sun dried tomatoes
- ¼ sliced shallot
- 10 basic leaves
- Salt (as per requirement)
- ½ cup Fairly grated Reggiano cheese

**Directions:**

Set the oven to preheat at 425F. Cover the baking tray with tomatoes, Brussels sprouts and garlic while drizzling it with oil and a pinch of salt and set it in the oven. Let the mixture be baked for about 30 minutes. During this time, boil the pasta in a utensil. Sauté shallots in a skillet for about 4 minutes and if preferred, introduce anchovies in it to brighten up the flavor. Now add the roasted mixture in the pan along with the pasta. Toss and enjoy.

5. **Sun-dried tomato pesto pasta**
   *Preparation time*: 10 minutes I *Cooking time*: 15-20 minutes I
   *Servings*: 4

**Ingredients:**

- 12 ounces Penne pasta
- 2 Cloves of garlic
- 1 Sun dried tomato in an olive oil jar
- 1 cup/freshly packed Basil leaves
- 1/2 cup finely shredded Parmesan
- Ground black pepper and salt

## Directions:

Bring the pasta to be boiled in a pot and set it aside after draining 3/4ᵗʰ of the liquid. On the other hand, place sun-dried tomatoes along with garlic, oil, pepper and salt in a blender and blend it intermittently until the tomatoes get fairly slashed. Now add up the blended mixture in a skillet and toss it with Parmesan cheese. Introduce pasta into the pan, toss it and enjoy the eternal flavor.

### 6. Creamy Tuscan Chicken
*Preparation time*: 10 minutes I ***Cooking time***: 15 minutes I ***Servings***: 6

## Ingredients:

- 2 tbsp. Olive oil
- Skinless/1.5 pounds sliced chicken breasts
- 1 cup heavy cream
- 1-2 tsp garlic powder
- 1/2 cup Parmesan cheese
- 1 cup Chopped spinach
- 1/2-1 cup sun-dried tomatoes
- 1 tsp Italian seasoning

## Directions:

In a large pot, cook chicken for a good time of 10 to 15 minutes until each of the side has properly been cooked and turned brown. Set the cooked chicken aside, introduce broth (chicken), Parmesan cheese, heavy cream and Italian seasoning in a skillet and toss it until the batter starts to condense. Place sun-dried tomatoes along with spinach and let the mixture simmer so that the spinach gets sagged. Mix chicken with the paste and add few pinches of garlic powder to enhance the flavor.

### 7. Chicken thigh with garlic and rosemary

*Preparation time*: 5 minutes | *Cooking time*: 30 minutes | *Servings*: 4 persons

**Ingredients:**

- Skinless/6 Chicken bone-in thighs
- 4 tbsp. olive oil
- 3 tbsp. fresh rosemary

- 4 minced cloves of garlic
- Ground pepper and salt (as required)
- 1 cup grape tomatoes

### Directions:

Place skinless chicken in a skillet and toss it with salt and pepper. Now after setting the chicken aside, add garlic and rosemary in a heated skillet containing olive oil and stir it for good amount of 1 minute until it turns aromatic. Introduce chicken into the pan while tossing it for 10 minutes and just before it is about to be cooked, add sun-dried tomatoes while whisking it for about 5 to 10 minutes. Serve chicken with rice or pasta depending on your choice and enjoy the delicious food.

### 8. One-pot beef with broccoli

*Preparation time*: 20 minutes | *Cooking time*: 25 minutes | *Servings*: 6 persons

Ingredients:

- 2 pounds of beef
- 1.5 cup hot water
- 4 cup broccoli
- 4 tbsp. soy sauce
- 2 tbsp. sesame oil

- 4 tsp corn starch
- 2 tbsp. brown sugar
- Olive oil and salt (as required)
- 3 cloves of garlic

### Directions:

Place all the liquid sauces in a mixing bowl and mix it thoroughly. Cook beef in a pan until it turns brown and when cooked, add the mixture of sauce into it. Bring the mixture to simmer while adding the vegetables into the skillet. Just when the vegetables and the beef turn tender, serve the dish alongside rice and enjoy the meal.

9.  **Vegan chickpea shakshuka**
    *Preparation time: 5 minutes I Cooking time: 25 minutes I Servings: 2 persons*

**Ingredients:**

- 2 tbsp. olive oil
- 1 bell pepper

- 2 cloves of garlic
- canned/400gram/1 cooked chickpeas
- Salt, basil leaves, thyme (as required)

- 1 onion
- 400 grams/1 sliced tomato
- 2 tbsp. tomato paste
- Canned olives

- Black pepper, rosemary, chili powder (to taste)

**Directions:**

Add the chopped vegetables, i.e. onion, bell peppers and cloves of garlic, into a heated pan. Sauté the added ingredients for at least 5-6 minutes until it turns soft and translucent. Introduce sun-dried tomatoes along with the tomato paste and the mentioned spices (rosemary, thyme, chili powder, salt) by bringing the mixture to be seethed. Add the dried chickpeas to the prepared sauce and stir it for 20 straight minutes so that it absorbs the flavor. Add olives to the pan and basil leaves for garnishing. Bon appetite!

## 10. Steak with lemon mashed potatoes

*Preparation time*: 10 minutes I *Cooking time*: 20 minutes **Servings**: 4 people

**Ingredients:**

- 1-1.5 pounds Yukon potatoes
- 1 cup frozen peas
- 2 sliced shallots
- 1-2 pounds/2 strips each thickening about ¾ strips of chicken/beef steak

- 2-3 tbsp. olive oil
- 2 tbsp./2 tsp respectively lemon juice and zest
- unsalted/1-1.5 tbsp. Butter
- Salt and pepper (to taste)

**Directions:**

Set the oven to 450F to preheat it. Now introduce the gold, peeled potatoes into the pot along with a cold water. Let the potato be boiled for about 15 minutes and just before it has been cooked, add peas to the pot in the final 5 minutes. After draining the liquid from the pot, add lemon zest and juice to it and mash it finely. On the other hand, cook the steak to your desired wellness and set it aside. To prepare the sauce, add sliced shallots into the skillet and transfer butter, salt and pepper, including wine to enhance the flavor to your preference. Serve the mashed potato with the respective prepared sauce and steak. Now enjoy!

## 11. Easy baked chicken for heartburn

*Preparation time*: 15 minutes I *Cooking time*: 45-50 minutes I **Servings**: 4 persons

**Ingredients:**

- Skinless/4 Chicken breasts
- 3 tbsp. shredded Parmesan cheese
- 1 cup bread crumbs

- 4 tbsp. olive oil
- Salt and ground black pepper (to taste)
- Italian seasoning (to taste)

## Directions:

Set the oven to 400F. In a mixture bowl, add shredded Parmesan cheese along with bread crumbs and the spices to coat the chicken breast. Pat the chicken breasts with traces of olive oil and introduce it into the prepared concoction of bread crumbs. Line up the patted, coated chicken breasts on the baking tray and set it aside to be baked for about 40 minutes. Bon appetite!

### 12. Chickpeas Hummus

*Preparation time*: 10 minutes I *Cooking time*: 10 minutes I *Servings*: 1.5 cups/6 people

## Ingredients:

- 1 cup chickpeas, canned or cooked
- 1 minced garlic
- 2 tbsp. olive oil
- Tahini and salt (to taste)

- 1/4 cup lemon juice
- 1/2 tsp cumin
- 3 tbsp. water

## Directions:

In a blender or a food processor, add tahini paste and the cup of chickpeas. Once blended for 1 minute, add olive oil, salt, and water along with cumin and minced garlic to the processor and blend it for another good 5 minutes. Add chickpeas into the blender and process it for about 2 minutes. To maintain the consistency, add water into the hummus until it reaches the desired texture.

### 13. Banana sorbet

*Preparation time: 5 minutes I **Cooking time**: 0 minutes I **Servings**: 1 person*

**Ingredients:**

- 1 ripe bananas
- ½ tbsp. chocolate chips
- 1tbsp. caramel syrup

**Directions:**

Once you pare banana a day before you have to prepare the sorbet, carve it down and store it in freezer. The very next day, grab the frozen, sliced bananas and introduce it in the blender along with any other ingredient (chocolate chips, caramel syrup, thawed chocolate) of your choice. Blend it and enjoy the moment all yourself or freeze it for consuming it later on.

### 14. Chicken with butternut squash

*Preparation time: 30 minutes I **Cooking time**: 30 minutes I **Servings**: 2-4 persons*

**Ingredients:**

- 4-6 tbsp. butter
- 1 lb. or pound butternut squash cut into cubes
- 4 ounces green beans
- 1 tsp paprika
- 1 tsp cloves of garlic crumbled
- 1/4 cup whole flour
- Skinless, boneless/1 pound chicken breasts
- Oregano, salt (to taste)

**Directions:**

Set the oven to be preheated at about 400F. Cover the baking tray with a sheet of aluminum foil or parchment. Now, in order to prepare butternut squash, cut the top portion of it while holding its base and cutting it into fine 2 pieces. Use a peeler to scrape off the covering from the butternut squash. Remove the seeds within and cut it into slices. When done, combine all the other ingredients along with the butternut squash and skinless chicken breasts. Toss the spices in it and place it down on the baking sheet. Set it aside to be baked for around 1 hour. Increase the heat in the oven to 450 degree Fahrenheit so that the chicken gets perfectly cooked inside and out. For brightening up the flavor, add thyme, oregano and paprika over and serve it hot.

### 15. Grilled pesto chicken

*Preparation time*: 60 minutes I *Cooking time*: 30 minutes I *Servings*: 4-6 persons

**Ingredients:**

- 1 cup pesto
- 1/4 cup Vinegar
- Skinless, boneless/2 pounds chicken breasts
- 1 tsp sugar
- 1 tsp salt

**Directions:**

To marinate the chicken effectively and evenly, take a ziplock bag and place the boneless/skinless chicken breast in it along with vinegar, pesto, sugar and salt inside. Shake it thoroughly so that the chicken breasts get marinated consistently. Set the zip locked bag aside in a refrigerator for about 2 hours. Now, to grill the chicken breast, preheat the oven or the open-air grate and place the marinated chicken upon it so that it gets equally cooked on both sides for good lot of 10 to 15 minutes. To let the chicken, absorb the flavor, let it sit aside for 5 minutes before shredding it on. Meanwhile, if one wants to cook it indoors, a skilled or a non-stick pan can be utilized to prepare the savory dish.

## 16. Bake potato & bacon

**Preparation time:** *30 minutes* | ***Cooking time****: 14 minutes* |
***Servings:*** *4*

**Ingredients:**

- 4 Idaho potatoes
- 2 tablespoons of extra virgin olive oil
- For filling:
- 6-8 pieces of bacon
- ½ cup sour cream
- 1 cup shredded cheddar cheese

- Salt and black pepper to taste
- 
- 
- 2 green onions finely chopped
- 1 cup shredded cheddar cheese
- 

**Directions:**

First of all, preheat the oven to 375F. Cook the bacon until golden and crisp out, cut it into small pieces and set aside until you are ready to use it. Wash the potatoes well to scrub all dust and dry them well before seasoning them, then poke the potatoes with a knife at 6 to 7 different places so filled steam will not allow them to burst. Drizzle potatoes with 2 tablespoons of the extra-virgin olive oil and season with salt and pepper to taste then bake them in the oven for 60 to 90 minutes. After baking mash, the opening of potatoes with a fork and fill it with cheese and bake again for 10 minutes until cheese gets melted. Garnish it with onions, sour cream and bacon. Enjoy!

## 17. Red onion chicken with rice

**Preparation time:** *60 minutes* | **Cooking time:** *35 minutes* |
**servings:** *4*

**Ingredients:**

- 1 pinch black pepper
- 2 boneless chicken breast
- 1 tbsp. fresh coriander

- 1 tbsp. sunflower oil
- 300 ml water
- 1 cinnamon stick

- 2 tbsp. curry powder
- 85g frozen peas

- 1 large red onion
- 1 tbsp. fresh mint

- 1 tbsp. raisin
- 4 tbsp. low fat natural yogurt
- 100g basmati rice
- 1 pinch salt

**Directions:**

Preheat the oven to 190F. Brush oil over the chicken and pepper it with curry powder. After tossing the onion slices in a roasting tin, add chicken over it and place it into the oven to cook for 30 minutes. Meanwhile, crisp onion separately in a pan. Boil rice in water until tender by adding 1 cinnamon stick and a pinch of salt and add peas to cook for 10 to 12 minutes. To serve, place rice on plate, add chicken, and sprinkle the onions as a topping. Add mint and coriander and serve with yogurt.

## 18. Bean and chicken sausages stew

*Preparation time:* 20 minutes | *Cooking time:* 20 minutes | *Servings:* 5

**Ingredients:**

- 2 tbsp. olive

- 3 chopped garlic cloves
- 1 chopped onion
- 1 Yellow capsicum
- 1 Red capsicum
- 6 cooking sausages

- 1½ tsp sweet smoked paprika
- 2 chopped celery
- 1 ½ Kg chopped tomatoes
- 1 chicken stock cube
- 400g can of beans
- 1 tbsp. fresh coriander

**Direction:**

Have oil in a pan and fry onions for 5 minutes, then add all chopped vegies yellow and red capsicum, celery sticks and cook for 5 minutes. Then add sausages to fry for 5 more minutes. After that, add chicken and water and cook for 10 minutes. Add garlic, smoked paprika, and cumin to cook until all aromas came out. Add tomato paste and thyme, then add chicken cubes and stir it, now keep it on the stove for 40 minutes. Afterwards, add beans and cook for more 5 minutes. Then season with black pepper. Now serve.

## 19. Brown sugar meatloaf

*Preparation time:* 10 - 15 minutes | *Cooking time:* 90 minutes | *Servings:* 5

**Ingredients:**

- ½ cup packed brown sugar
- ½ cup ketchup
- 2 eggs
- ¼ teaspoon ground black pepper
- ¼ teaspoon ground ginger
- 1½ pounds lean ground beef
- ¾ cup milk
- 1 ½ teaspoons salt
- 1 small onion
- ¾ cup cracker crumbs

**Directions:**

Let preheat oven at 350 degrees. Brush the oil over the loaf pan. Now add beef sprinkle brown sugar, pour ketchup and toss well. In a separate bowl ass milk, eggs, salt, black pepper, ginger, and make a fine blend. Apply the mixture over beef evenly. Toss the beef into cracker crumb and set in pan. Sprinkle onion and bake it for 80 to 85 minutes or until cooked and juicy. Enjoy with ketchup or a sauce of your choice.

## 20. Cocktail Meatballs

*Preparation time:* 15 minutes | *Cooking time:* 90 minutes | *Servings:* 5

**Ingredients:**

- 1 pound lean ground beef
- 1 egg
- ½ cup bread crumbs
- 2 tablespoons water
- 3 tablespoons crushed onion

**Directions:**

Preheat oven at 375 degrees for 20 minutes. In a mixing bowl, add all ingredients beef, egg, water, bread crumbs and onions. Mix them well and take a small quantity with spoon and make round balls. Take a baking pan and set parchment paper with oil grease. Set the meat round balls into the baking try and bake for 20 to 25 minutes or until cooked and turned brown. Serve with sauce, ketchup or anything you love. Enjoy!

## 21. Grilled corn cob with lime

**Preparation time:** *15 minutes | Cooking time: 25 minutes | Servings: 4*

**Ingredients:**

- ½ cup butter
- 1 zest lime
- 4 corns sticks
- 1 can chipotle peppers
- Salt to taste

**Directions:**

Take a grill and heat at a low medium flame. Grease it with oil. Take a bowl and add butter, chipotle peppers, lime zest, and salt and mix until combine. Let the mixture set aside for few minutes. Now toss the mixture over the corncobs and let them grill for 20 to 25 minutes until it cooked well. Every 10 minutes, change the side of corncobs over the grill. Serve immediately!

## 22. Mexican baked fish

**Preparation time:** *20 minutes | Cooking time: 15 minutes | Servings: 5*

**Ingredients:**

- 1 cup of salsa
- 1 ½ shredded cheddar cheese
- 1 ½ cup avocado
- 2 fish fillets
- ½ cup crushed corn chips
- ¼ cup sour cream
- 1 ½ pound cod

**Directions:**

Preheat oven to 400 degrees and set the baking tray by greasing it and setting it aside. Put the fish fillets on baking tray and sprinkle shredded cheese, corn chips and salsa over it. Remember, the topping must be with corn chips. Put into oven and bake for 15 to 20 minutes or until cooked. Now remove and add avocado slices and bake for more 5 minutes. Now serve with sour cream.

## 23. Sesame noodles with chicken

*Preparation time:* 5 minutes | *Cooking time:* 20 minutes | *Servings:* 5

### Ingredients:

- 1 pack of spaghetti
- 2 scallions
- 1 tbsp. garlic paste
- 2 tbsp. soya sauce
- 400-gram chicken breast
- 1 cup peas
- 3 tbsp. sesame oil
- 2 tsp. ginger paste
- 1 tsp. brown sugar
- 2 tbsp. ketchup
- 1 cup chopped carrot
- 3 tbsp. sesame seeds

### Directions:

Boil spaghetti as per package instruction. Drain and rinse then shift into a big bowl. Mix sesame oil, scallions, garlic, ginger, and sugar in a separate bowl. Heat over a low or medium fire until it sizzles and cook for 2 minutes. Now, turn off the flame and stir in ketchup and soy sauce. Now, add crushed and chopped carrots and shredded cheese into noodles then put it into a pan and serve!

## 24. Salmon tacos with pineapple salsa

*Preparation time:* 12 minutes | *Cooking time:* 15 minutes | *Servings:* 5

### Ingredients:

- 1 pound salmon
- ¾ tsp. salt
- 5 cups mixed coleslaw
- 6-inch corn tortillas
- Chopped fresh cilantro
- 1 tsp. chili powder
- 2 tbsp. olive oil
- ½ lemon juice
- ¾ cup pineapple salsa
- Hot sauce to serve

## Directions:

Place a baking sheet with foil where salmon will be below up to 3 to 4 inch. Preheat broiler until it gets completely hot. Line a baking dish with aluminum foil. Place salmon and bake one side until it gets browned and bake another afterwards to make it brown too. All fillet will take about 10 minutes to reach that point. Now sprinkle chili powder and ¼ tsp salt and place it back in the oven for 2 more minutes to let absorb inside with spices. Next, toss coleslaw onto a pan with 1 tsp. salt and 1 tbsp. olive oil. Get the salmon out and divide it among tortillas. For topping, use salsa and garnish with cilantro and serve!

## 25. Bake bacon French toast

> **Preparation time:** *15 minutes* | **Cooking time:** *30 minutes* | **Servings:** *5*

## Ingredients:

- 8 cups cubed bread
- 2 cups of milk
- ½ cup packed brown sugar
- 1 cup shredded cheddar cheese
- 8 eggs
- ½ tsp. cinnamon
- 1 pound bacon

## Directions:

Place a baking dish on slap and put bread greased with oil under butter paper. Just line up every ingredient over bread, i.e. eggs, milk brown sugar, bacon, cinnamon, and cheese. Freeze it into the refrigerator overnight. Remove it from the fridge the next day before 30 minutes to cook. Preheat oven to bake at 375F. and bake it for 1 hour until a knife goes into it and comes out clean. Hold on 10 minutes to serve as it gets to be hot.

## 26. Farro salad with grilled steak
**Preparation time:** *10 minutes* | **Cooking time:** *10 minutes* |
*Servings: 2*

**Ingredients:**

- 1 can farro
- 5 tbsp. olive oil
- 2 cups of corn
- ¼ balsamic vinegar
- 2 medium bell peppers
- 500 grams of beef
- 1 cup kale leaves

**Directions:**

Cook farro as per instruction on the package is given. Toss bell peppers
in 2 tbsp. olive oil. Grill steaks and sprinkle pepper and cook until
doneness of beef. Grill the beef and stuff with all remaining crunchy
peppers to taste. Toss farro with pepper. Add corn, kale leaves, balsamic
vinegar, salt to taste and olive oil. Now serve with farro.

## 27. Chicken breast with tomato pesto
**Preparation time:** *15 minutes* | **Cooking Time:** *90 minutes* |
*Servings: 5*

**Ingredients:**

- 4 chicken breasts
- 1 cup Dijon mustard
- 15 ounce roasted
  tomatoes
- Salt and pepper to taste
- ½ cup pesto sauce
- ¼ cup red wine vinegar
- ¼ cup chicken broth

**Directions:**

Let preheat oven for 15 minutes on 375 F. Grease baking dish with
cooking spray and spread all chicken breast pieces. Then pour tomatoes
into and season with salt and pepper, pour red wine and other
remaining ingredients. Remember to place a foil underneath and cook
for 80 to 85 minutes. Serve it with tomato sauce itself for a yummy and
delicious meal.

## 28. Sheet Pan Nachos with Veggies

*Preparation time: 1 hour | Cooking time: 30 - 40 minutes | Servings: 5*

**Ingredients:**

- 1 tsp. olive oil
- 1 clove garlic
- 1 ½ tsp. sea salt
- ½ tsp. ground cumin
- 1 cup green and red salsa
- 1 avocado
- 15 oz. unsalted pinto beans
- 4 tbsp. fresh lime juice
- 1 tsp. chili powder
- 16 ounce tortilla chips
- ½ cup cilantro leaves
- 2 ounce cheddar cheese

**Directions:**

Have a frying pan and fry garlic in oil add all seasonings and veggies and stir fry until the color changes. Now set it aside. Separately, the toss pan get smoke to all of the seasonings. Now mix both well. Top with tortilla chips, cilantro and a ripe avocado. Spread cheese on top of everything and bake on preheated oven for 20 minutes.

## 29. Stir fry vegetables with teriyaki

*Preparation time: 30 minutes | Cooking time: 40 minutes | Servings: 4*

**Ingredients:**

- 2 tbsp. olive oil
- 3 cloves crushed garlic
- 2 cup carrot
- ¾ cup roasted salted cashews
- 1 cup green onions
- 2 cup brown rice
- For sauce:
- 1 can pineapple
- 2 tbsp. honey
- 1 tbsp. chia seeds
- 1 medium onion
- 1 tbsp. ginger paste
- 2 bell peppers
- 1 large broccoli chopped
- 1 ½ cup peas
- 1 cup soya sauce
- 1 tbsp. rice vinegar

## Directions:

For teriyaki, have oil in a toss pan on medium flame and throw onion onto it. Now add ginger garlic paste and fry well. Known mixer aroma is about to spread. Pour all veggies and cook till fry. Even pour cashews though. For sauce, first have a pineapple with juice in a pan on a low medium flame. Twist a spoon until the juice is released. Now, you need to add honey soy sauce and rice vinegar while continuously stirring with a spoon. Add seeds into the sauce. Now, pour out the sauce you need and veggies to eat. Mix in separate bowl and enjoy!

## 30. Quinoa Tacos

*Preparation time:* 20 minutes | *Cooking time:* 30 minutes | *Servings:* 5

## Ingredients:

- 1 tbsp. olive oil
- 2 garlic cloves
- 1 ½ cup Beans
- 1 tsp green chili
- 1 cup quinoa
- 1 cup frozen corn
- 1 onion
- 1 tbsp. cilantro
- 2 cups chicken broth
- 3 tomatoes
- Mixed spices
- Tortillas

## Directions:

Preheat oven for 10 minutes at 375F. Now grease baking dish with cooking spray and add in the quinoa. Pour all ingredients over it one at a time, including yellow onion, and the other veggies. Now in a pan on medium flame, just fry boiled beans, frozen corn. Now pour it onto fish. Season with all the spices, including the cumin, paprika and other ingredients to your preference. Bake it in the oven for 30 minutes. Top it with tortillas and serve

# Chapter 7: Recipes for Snacks & Desserts

### 1. Blueberry cherry chip

*Preparation time*: 15 minutes | *Cooking time*: 40 minutes | *Servings*: 8

**Ingredients:**

- 1 cup oat meal
- ½ cup macadamia nuts
- 3 tbsp. butter
- 1 tsp cinnamon
- 1/8 tsp salt
- 2 cup blueberries, frozen
- 1/3 cup whole wheat flour
- 2 tbsp. coconut oil
- 2 tbsp. honey
- ¼ tsp nutmeg
- 4 cup cherry frozen

**Directions:**

First of all, preheat oven at 375 degrees, and set the baking dish by greasing with butter. Take a bowl and add oatmeal, flour, nuts and mix well. Now in a pan add coconut oil, butter, honey, cinnamon, nutmeg and salt. Stir the mixture on low flame until butter melt and mixture well combine. Cook it for 3 minutes, after that pour it on the oatmeal mixture and stir well. Set the berries and cherries in a dish and pour mixture over them with spoon. Bake them for 35 to 40 minutes or until crispy. Serve when cool down.

## 2. Baked apple with tahini raisin filling

*Preparation time*: 15 minutes I *Cooking time*: 30 minutes I
*Servings*: 4

**Ingredients:**

- 4 apples
- 1 cup apple juice
- 1/3 cup pecans
- Nutmeg as per taste
- ¾ cup water boiling
- ¾ cup tahini
- 3 tbsp. raisins
- ¼ tsp cinnamon
- Vanilla as per taste

**Directions:**

Set the baking dish with oil grease and heat oven at 375 degrees. Cut the apples from the center to remove the core and set them in baking dish. Take a small bowl, add tahini, apple juice, cinnamon, nutmeg, and vanilla and mix them together. Now fill the center core of apples with the mixture. Pour the boiling water in baking dish, apple juice over the apples, and bake for 30 minutes. After that, remove from the oven and serve warm.

## 3. Pear banana nut muffins

*Preparation time*: 30 minutes I *Cooking time*: 20 minutes I
*Servings*: 12

**Ingredients:**

- 1 pear
- 1 cup whole wheat flour
- 1 tbsp. flaxseed
- 1 tsp baking powder
- 1 tsp cinnamon
- ¼ tsp salt
- 1/3 cup almond milk
- 2 tsp vanilla
- 2 tbsp. pear nectar
- 1 cup oats
- 3 tbsp. maple syrup
- ½ baking soda
- ¼ tsp cardamom
- 2 eggs
- 2 tbsp. butter
- 1 medium banana

- 1 cup walnuts, chopped

## Directions:

Preheat oven to 375F, set the muffin cup with parchment paper, and set aside. In a pan, add pear nectar and pear and boil over medium heat. When it starts to simmer, then reduce the heat and cook until smooth. Let it cool. In a bowl, add flour, oats, flaxseeds, baking soda, baking powder, cinnamon, cardamom, and salt and mix well. In another bowl, add the peach syrup, eggs, almond milk, butter, and vanilla to whisk well. Add banana and after mixing, pour it on the dry ingredients. Fold them well and pour into the muffin cups. Bake them for the 20 minutes or until well cooked and turn brown. Remove and let them cool down before serving.

### 4. Berry banana slush

*Preparation time*: 5 minutes I *Cooking time*: 5 minutes I *Servings*: 2

### Ingredients:

- 2 banana
- Ice cubes if required
- 200 g frozen berries

## Directions:

Take a blender and pour the mixed berries inside, including blueberries, strawberries and raspberries and blend them well until turns to a combined slush. Add ice for if you'd like to increase the slushy consistency. In serving cups, add the banana cubes, and pour the berry slush on them. Serve the chill and yummy banana berry slush.

### 5. Sticky toffee pudding

***Preparation time****: 25 minutes I **Cooking time***: 1 hour I
***Servings****: 4*

**Ingredients:**

- 175 g dates, dried
- 1 tbsp. vanilla extract
- 85g flour

- 150 ml maple syrup
- 2 eggs

**Directions:**

Preheat oven at 180 degrees. Take a pan add water and pour dates cook on low flame for 5 to 6 minutes. Add the dates and water into blender and pulse until turn smooth. Add maple syrup and vanilla extract and blend again. Pour the mixture into a bowl, now whisk egg into separate bowl. In dates mixture add flour, egg and fold them well until well combined. Take pudding pan and pour maple syrup into the base, now pour the mixture on it and bake for at least an hour. After that, transfer it to the serving plate, dress it with maple syrup and serve.

### 6. Baked apple with cinnamon & ginger

***Preparation time****: 10 minutes I **Cooking time***: 40 minutes I
***Servings****: 4*

**Ingredients:**

- 4 apples
- ½ tsp cinnamon
- 50 g muscovado sugar
- 4 scoops vanilla ice cream
  for serving

- 2 ginger, chopped
- 4 prunes, chopped
- 1 tbsp. butter

**Directions:**

Preheat oven to 200F. Cut the quarter of each apple and set them into a baking dish. Take a bowl, add ginger, cinnamon, sugar, prunes and butter, and mix well. Pour the mixture over the apples and put the butter on each apple top. Bake them for 35 minutes or until cooked well. Remove and serve the hot baked cinnamon apple with a scoop of vanilla ice cream.

### 7. Chocolate muffin with chocolate custard

*Preparation time: 10 minutes I **Cooking time**: 10 minutes I Servings: 6*

**Ingredients:**

- 1 tbsp. cocoa powder
- ½ tsp baking soda
- 100 ml skimmed milk
- 2 tbsp. sunflower oil
- 25g dark chocolate

- 100 g raising flour
- 50 g caster sugar
- 1 egg
- 150g low fat custard

**Directions:**

Preheat the oven and set the muffin tray by greasing it with oil. In a large bowl, add flour, cocoa powder, sugar, soda, and mix well. In another bowl, whisk eggs, milk, oil and mix together. Pour the mixture on dry ingredients and make a fine batter. Now, pour the mixture with the help of a spoon on the muffins tray and bake for 10 to 15 minutes or until cooked and turned brown. While they are in the oven, pour custard into a pan and add dark chocolate into it or stir until combined and smooth. When the muffins are done, put it onto the serving plate, pour hot custard over it, and serve hot.

### 8. Lighter Apple & pear pie

*Preparation time*: 20 minutes I *Cooking time*: 40 minutes I
*Servings*: 6

## Ingredients:

- 6 apples
- 1 lemon juice & zest
- 1 tsp mix spice
- 4 pastry sheets
- 25g almond

- 4 pears
- 3 tbsp. syrup
- 1 tbsp. corn flour
- 4 tsp rapeseed oil

## Directions:

Take a pan, add apples and pears with water, syrup, lemon and mixed spices, and cook for 5 minutes. Now, remove the fruit and pour it into a pie dish and cook the remainder for another 5 minutes. Mash the remaining fruits into a mixture until smooth and until the syrup is thick in consistency. Cook that syrup for another 4 to 5 minutes and then pour it into a pie dish. Set the pastry sheets in the dish and brush oil on the top. Bake it for 30 minutes in a preheated oven at 180 degrees, until it turns brown and is cooked. Serve immediately!

### 9. Peach & blueberry yogurt cake

*Preparation time*: 20 minutes I *Cooking time*: 1 hour I
*Servings*: 10

## Ingredients:

- 1 ½ cup all-purpose flour
- ½ tsp baking soda
- 1 cup sugar
- ½ tsp vanilla
- 2 peaches, sliced
- 1 tsp sugar

- 1 tsp baking powder
- 2 oz. butter
- 2 eggs
- ½ cup yogurt
- 6 oz. blueberries

**Directions:**

Grease the baking pan with parchment paper and set aside, preheat the oven to 350 degrees. Take a bowl, add flour, baking powder and soda. In a separate bowl, whisk eggs, butter, and sugar until fluffy. Now add vanilla extract and Greek yogurt and continue beating until well combined and the texture becomes smooth. Pour the mixture into a flour bowl and mix until well combined. Pour the batter into baking pan, set the slices of peach and sprinkle blueberries with sugar. Bake it for 30 to 35 minutes or until golden brown. When baking is done, let it cool down for 30 minutes and then serve with the yogurt topping.

### 10. Dark chocolate cheese bar

*Preparation time: 15 minutes I Cooking time: 1 hour I Servings: 12*

**Ingredients:**

- 1 cup cracker crumbs
- ¼ cup cocoa powder
- 2 tbsp. honey
- 2 to 3 tbsp. almond milk
- ¼ cup coconut flour
- 8 tbsp. cream cheese
- 1 tsp vanilla extract
- 1/3 cup dark chocolate chips
- 1 tsp coconut oil

**Directions:**

Set up a tray with the parchment paper and set it aside. Take a bowl and add graham cracker crumbs, coconut flour, and cocoa powder, and add them into a mixture. Then pour honey, vanilla extract and cream cheese. Mix them well to turn then into a fine dough. Gradually add the almond milk to make the dough soft and do not let it dry. When it's done, set it into a baking pan with the help of spatula. In a small bowl, add chocolate chips and coconut oil and set it into the microwave until melted and smooth. Pour the chocolate over the batter and set it evenly. Now put the tray into the fridge for some time until the ingredients set well. Now serve the fine dark chocolate cheese bar.

### 11. Skinny chocolate chip cheesecake bar

*Preparation time: 15 minutes I **Cooking time**: 35 minutes I Servings: 16*

**Ingredients:**

- ¾ cup graham cracker crumbs
- 8 oz. cream cheese
- 2 eggs
- 2 tbsp. flour
- 2 tbsp. vanilla extract
- 2 tbsp. butter
- ¾ cup Greek yogurt
- ¼ cup sugar
- 1 tbsp. lemon juice
- ½ cup chocolate chips

**Directions:**

Preheat the oven to 350F and set the baking tray by setting parchment paper and set aside. In a blender, add cracker crumbs and pour butter to blend well. Transfer the mixture into a baking tray and set it with a spatula and bake for 8 to 10 minutes. In a mixer, add cream cheese and beat for a minute. Now add yogurt, egg, sugar, and flour and mix until smooth. Add the lemon juice and mix well. Now pour the mixture into a bowl and add chocolate chips and fold them well. Cover the baked crust with the cream cheese filling and bake for 20 to 25 minutes until cooked. After that, let it cool down and serve hot or chilled.

### 12. Frozen fruit skewers

*Preparation time: 30 minutes I **Cooking time**: 0 I Servings: 12*

**Ingredients:**

- ¼ of watermelon, cubed
- ½ pineapple, cubed
- ½ cantaloupe, cubed
- 1 cup grapes

- 6 oz. blueberries
- 4 oz. chocolate chips
- 2 to 3 banana, sliced

**Directions:**

Take the fruits and cut them in evenly into cubes. Thread the fruit alternatively on the skewers. Now cover the skewers with a plastic sheet and put in them in the refrigerator until ready to serve. In a bowl, add chocolate chips and melt in a microwave for 2 to 3 minutes until smooth. Let the chocolate cool down a bit. Remove the fruit skewers and drizzle the melted chocolate over the fruit skewers. Now put it into refrigerator and let it freeze. Serve frozen fruit skewer immediately!

### 13. Whole wheat chocolate cake donuts

*Preparation time: 5 minutes | Cooking time: 15 minutes | Servings: 6*

**Ingredients:**

- ¾ cup almond milk
- 1 cup whole wheat flour
- 2 tsp cocoa powder
- ½ tsp baking soda
- ½ tbsp. flax seed
- 1 cup sugar, powdered
- 1 tbsp. milk
- 1 tsp lemon juice
- 2 tbsp. sugar
- ½ tsp baking powder
- ½ tsp salt
- 2 tbsp. oil
- 1 tsp vanilla extract

**Directions:**

Preheat oven at 350F and set the donut baking tray. In a small bowl, mix the almond milk with lemon juice and set aside for 5 minutes. In a bowl, add flour, flaxseed, sugar, cocoa powder, baking powder, baking soda, salt, oil ,and mix them well. Now pour the almond milk and lemon mixture into it and mix it until combined. Pour the batter over the donut baking tray and bake for 10 to 13 minutes or until fluffy and cooked. Remove them and let them cool down. Sprinkle powdered sugar or milk. Serve immediately or store for later use.

### 14. Blueberry and cream dessert

*Preparation time*: *30 minutes I* ***Cooking time***: *15 minutes I*
***Servings***:

**Ingredients:**

- 12 oz. blueberries, frozen
- 2 tbsp. cornstarch
- 1 tbsp. lemon juice
- 2/3 cup dried milk
- 1 ½ heavy cream

- 2 tbsp. sugar
- ¼ cup water
- 16 oz. light cream cheese
- 2/3 cup granulated sugar
- 3 tbsp. powdered sugar

**Directions:**

Take a pan and add water, blueberries, sugar, cornstarch and lemon juice. Bring it to a boil and simmer for 5 to 7 minutes over a medium flame. Let it cool down to room temperature. For the cake and cream layer, take a blender, add cream cheese, milk, sugar and blend until smooth and creamy. Fold the cream cheese mixture with the cake cubes until well combined. Mix the heavy cream with sugar for the whipped cream until it turns soft and fluffy. In a serving cup, fill it with the mixture, and add blueberry syrup and another layer of cream cheese cake. After that, dress it with the whipped cream and put it in the refrigerator for 2 hours to set and chill it. Serve the chilled blueberry cream dessert.

### 15. Cream cheese lemon coffee cake

*Preparation time*: *20 minutes I* ***Cooking time***: *40 minutes I*
***Servings***: *16*

**Ingredients:**

- 8 oz. cream cheese
- 2 egg
- 1 ½ cup flour

- ¼ cup sugar
- 2 tsp lemon juice
- ½ tsp baking powder

- ¼ tsp baking soda
- ½ cup vegetable oil
- ½ cup Greek yogurt
- Powdered sugar for dust
- ¼ tsp salt
- ¾ cup granulated sugar
- 1 lemon zest

**Directions:**

Preheat oven to 350F and set the parchment paper in a baking try and grease it with oil. In a bowl, add cream cheese, sugar, egg and lemon juice, mix the ingredients until well combined and turn smooth. In another bowl, add flour, baking powder, baking soda and salt and mix them together. In blender, add egg, oil and sugar and blend until smooth. Add yogurt, lemon zest and lemon juice and make a fine mixture. After that, add the flour gradually into the mixture and continue mixing on a medium speed. When the mixture is well combined, pour it into a baking tray and set well. Pour the cream cheese mixture over it and set well. Bake it for 40 to 45 minutes or until cooked. Remove it from the oven and let it cool down. Cut into slices and serve.

### 16. Baked pears with walnuts and honey

*Preparation time: 5 minutes | Cooking time: 25 minutes | Servings: 4*

**Ingredients:**

- 2 pears
- ¼ tsp cinnamon
- Salt as per taste
- ¼ cup honey
- ¼ tsp vanilla extract
- ¼ cup walnuts

**Directions:**

First of all, preheat the oven to 400F and set the parchment paper into the baking tray and set aside. Slice the pear from the center with a knife and remove the seeds. Set the pears into a baking tray over parchment paper. In a bowl, add cinnamon, honey, salt and vanilla extract and mix well. With a spoon, pour the mixture over the pears evenly and bake for the 20 to 25 minutes. Remove when cooked well, then garnish with walnuts and honey over the pears and serve.

### 17. Apple baked chips

*Preparation time: 5 minute' I Cooking time: 1 hour, 20 minutes I Servings: 1 bowl*

**Ingredients:**

- 3 large apples
- 2 tsp sugar
- 1 tsp cinnamon
- 1tsp olive oil

**Directions:**

First of all, preheat the oven to 200F and set the baking tray with parchment paper and set it aside. With a sharp knife, cut the apple to remove its core from center and make round slices. Set the apple slices on parchment paper, spray olive oil, and apply cinnamon and sugar to each slice. Bake the apples for 40 minutes. Now remove and flip the side and add some cinnamon or cook again for 40 minutes. Let them become golden brown and crispy. Remove and let them cool. These can be stored for 3 days.

### 18. Banana, honey & peanut butter roll

*Preparation time: I Cooking time: I Servings:*

**Ingredients:**

- 1 flatbread
- ½ banana
- 1 tbsp. peanut butter
- ½ tbsp. honey

**Directions:**

Take banana and cut into slices. On a flatbread, spread the peanut butter with the help of knife and spread evenly. Place the banana chunks on top and pour some honey over top. Make a roll of the bread and cut the center in half. Serve with milk or enjoy plain for a snack.

### 19. Blueberry oatmeal Greek yogurt muffins

*Preparation time*: 10 minutes I *Cooking time*: 30 minutes I *Servings*: 6

**Ingredients:**

- 1 cup all-purpose flour
- 2 tsp baking powder
- 2 eggs
- 1/3 cup honey
- 2 tsp vanilla extract
- 1 cup oats
- ¼ tsp salt
- 1 cup plain yogurt
- ¼ cup milk
- 1 cup blueberries

**Directions:**

Preheat the oven to 350F and set the parchment paper into a muffin tray and set aside. Separate 1tbsp flour aside. In a bowl, add the rest of the flour, oats, baking powder and salt. In another bowl, whisk the eggs, yogurt, honey, milk and vanilla extract. After that, pour the flour into the mixture and fold them well until combined. Add blueberries into it and mix well. Pour the mixture into muffin cups evenly. Bake for 20 minutes or until golden and cooked. Take them out and let them cool. Sprinkle some flour or serve with a yogurt topping.

### 20. Caprese salad

*Preparation time: 5 minutes I Cooking time: 5 minutes I Servings: 1*

**Ingredients:**

- 1 tbsp. balsamic vinegar
- ½ tbsp. olive oil
- 1 ½ leaves of basil
- 1 tomato
- 1 oz. mozzarella
- Salt & pepper to taste

**Directions:**

Take the tomato, and wash and cut it into slices. In a medium bowl, add the tomato, vinegar, olive oil, salt and pepper and toss them well until combined. Now add mozzarella and mix well. Sprinkle some basil leaves on top and serve.

### 21. Chickpeas with white toast

*Preparation time: 5 minutes I Cooking time: 5 minutes I Servings: 1*

**Ingredients:**

- 1 slice of white bread
- 3 tbsp. grated carrot
- 1 lemon juice
- ¼ cup chickpeas, boiled
- 1 tsp olive oil
- Salt & pepper to taste

**Directions:**

Take a small bowl and add chickpeas and mash them with the help of a fork. Now, add olive oil, lemon juice, carrot chunks and salt or pepper to your taste. Mix them well until combined. Take a slice of toast and apply the mixture on the toast with a knife. Sprinkle some carrot on top and serve as a healthy snack.

### 22. Baked zucchini chips

*Preparation time*: 10 minutes I *Cooking time*: 2 hours I *Servings*: 1 bowl

**Ingredients:**

- 1 zucchini
- Salt to taste
- 2 tbsp. olive oil

**Directions:**

To begin, preheat the oven to 225F and set the parchment paper in a baking tray and set it aside. Take zucchini and cut it into round slices with 2 to 3 of thickness. Set the zucchini slices on the baking tray and cover it with a paper towel, set another layer and again cover it with a towel. It helps to absorb the extra moisture while baking. Press the zucchini slice well between a towel so the moisture will absorb. Now brush the olive oil on each slice and sprinkle some salt. Bake them in a preheated oven for 2 hours or until they turn brown or turn crispy. Serve when they cool down or store for up to 2 days.

### 23. White bean salad

*Preparation time*: 5 minutes I *Cooking time*: 5 minutes I *Servings*: 2

**Ingredients:**

- 1 cup white beans
- 1 tomato
- ½ lemon juice
- ¼ cup vinegar
- ½ cucumber
- Handful of dill
- 1 cup white beans
- Salt as per taste

**Directions:**

In a pan full of water, boil the white beans until soft and cooked. Now, drain out the water and set them aside. Wash the tomato and cucumber and cut it into cubes. Take a medium bowl and add cucumber, tomato, dill, lemon juice, vinegar and boiled white beans. Now mix them well. Sprinkle some salt as per your taste and toss to combine. Serve the refreshing white bean salad as a snack.

### 24. Banana pudding cookie

*Preparation time*: 5 minutes I *Cooking time*: 10 minutes I *Servings*: 12

## Ingredients:

- 3 bananas
- 1 egg
- 3 tablespoons unsalted butter
- 2/3 cup plain flour
- 1 teaspoon vanilla
- 3 tablespoons plain yogurt
- 1 teaspoon baking powder
- ¼ cup Sugar
- ¼ teaspoon salt
- 1 pack vanilla pudding mix

## Directions:

In a bowl, add mashed bananas and baking soda. Mix it well and set aside. Beat egg, and add cream, sugar, yogurt, and butter in it and whisk it. In another bowl, mix pudding mix, flour, and salt and add this mixture to the cream mixture and whisk well. In the end, add the banana mixture in it and combine well. Now, on the greased baking dish, scoop the batter in the form of cookies. Bake in for 10 minutes in the preheated oven on the temperature of 350F.

### 25. Vanilla cupcake

*Preparation time*: 10 minutes | *Cooking time*: 20 minutes | *Servings*: 12

## Ingredients:

- 2 cups flour
- ¾ cup sugar
- 2 eggs
- 1 teaspoon vanilla extract
- 1 teaspoon baking soda
- 1 cup milk
- ½ cup butter
- ½ teaspoon salt

## Directions:

Preheat the oven to 375F. Prepare the muffin tins with a liner. In a bowl, whisk butter and sugar and add eggs one by one. Add all the remaining items and mix well. Pour the batter in the muffin tins and bake it in the preheated oven for around 18 minutes and serve it.

### 26. White chocolate and strawberry tart

*Preparation time*: 15 minutes | *Cooking time*: 10 minutes | *Servings*: 2

## Ingredients:

- 5 teaspoon melted butter
- 1 cup ground shortbread cookies
- 3 tablespoons cream
- ¾ cup fresh sliced strawberries

- 1 1/3 cups melted butter
- 1 ½ cups grated white chocolate
- 2 tablespoons chocolate chips

## Directions:

Prepare a baking tray with a greased baking liner. Mix the crumble cookers and butter and pour it in the baking dish and press it properly from every side. Bake it for 10 minutes at a 350F temperature. Microwave the beaten cream for 20 seconds and add white chocolate in it and whisk. Pour this filling on the baked crust and add chocolate chips and strawberries on its top.

### 27. Baileys custard

*Preparation time*: 2 minutes / *Cooking time*: 10 minutes / *Servings*: 4

## Ingredients:

- 4 egg yolks
- 3 ½ cups cream
- ½ cup baileys can
- ¼ cup sugar
- 1 teaspoon vanilla extract
- ½ cup milk

## Directions:

Take a bowl and mix all the ingredients thoroughly. Now put it in a pot and cook over 90C temperature for approximately 10 minutes. You can serve it immediately or can serve it cold. For cooling it keep it in the refrigerator for some time and present it.

## 28. Mexican bean salad

**Preparation time**: *15 minutes I* **Chilling time**: *1-hour I* **Servings**: *8*

**Ingredients:**

- 15 ounce rinsed and drained black beans
- 1 chopped green bell pepper
- 1 chopped onion
- 1 chopped red bell pepper
- 15 ounce rinsed and drained kidney beans
- ½ cup olive oil
- 10 ounce cooked corn
- 2 tablespoons lemon juice
- 2 chicken breasts
- ½ cup vinegar
- 1 minced garlic
- 2 tablespoons sugar
- ½ tablespoon ground black pepper
- ½ tablespoon ground cumin
- 15 ounce rinsed and drained cannellini beans

## Directions:

Take a bowl and add all the wet ingredients. Mix them well and add the remaining ingredients in it. Whisk all the ingredients until they combine well. Put it in the refrigerator for an hour and serve.

## 29. Peanut butter no bake cookies

**Preparation time**: *10 minutes I* **Cooking time**: *1 hour I*
**Servings**: *14 cookies*

### Ingredients:

- ½ cup peanut butter
- 1/3 cup maple syrup
- ¼ cup milk
- ½ cup dark chocolate
- 1 banana
- 1 ½ cup quinoa flakes
- 1/8 tsp salt

### Directions:

Set the parchment paper into a baking tray and set it aside. In a bowl, add peanut butter and banana and mash well. Take a pan and add maple syrup or peanut butter and banana mixture to cook for 2 minutes until combined. Take off the flame and add quinoa flakes, milk, and salt and mix. Let the mixture cool down for about 10 minutes. Meanwhile, melt the dark chocolate in a microwave and fold it into the mixture. Use a scope and make round balls and then flatten them into the shape of cookies. Place the cookies over the parchment paper and leave them into refrigerator for 1 hour. Serve when set and chilled.

### 30. Cucumber roll ups

*Preparation time*: 5 minutes I *Cooking time*: 10 minutes I *Servings*: 12

**Ingredients:**

- 1 lb. tomatoes
- ½ onion
- 2 tbsp. olive oil
- 1 tbsp. honey
- ¼ tsp black pepper
- 1 cucumber
- 2 avocados
- 2 tbsp. vinegar
- ½ tsp salt

**Directions:**

Wash the tomatoes and cucumber and cut them with a knife. Slice the cucumber into long slices. Similarly, cut and mash the avocados. Take a bowl add the avocado mixture, tomatoes, olive oil, honey, salt, pepper, and vinegar. Mix them all together well and set aside. Take the cucumber slices and apply the mixture over them and then roll up the slices. Serve the cucumber roll ups as a snack and enjoy.

# Conclusion

Acid reflux is a stomach related or digestive disorder that creates irritation and a restless condition for a person. The main reason behind this issue is poor digestion, improper food intake, lack of sleep, and inactivity. An increase in obesity and other health complications can cause acid reflux. In this chronic disorder, a person feels heartburn and feels like their food is not properly being digested. Stomach acid and food reverse into the food canal that causes an inability to perform the task and continuous burp can affect a person's productivity as well.

As per the consultants, it is necessary to treat the acid reflux at the initial stage with food intake, exercise, and diet control by reducing the weight or following proper medication. It not treated well, then it may cause further health complications like cancer or ulcers as well. To get quick relief from acid reflux, it is necessary to adopt certain dietary changes like taking small meals instead of full meals, following an exercise routine, reducing citrus intake, limiting spicy and fried food intake, and reducing weight. At the initial stage of acid reflux, it can be treated and prevented with healthy and organic food choices. It also requires a proper medical checkup; this helps to find out how severe the problem is. Consulting doctors and taking their advice for the treatment and precautions is a necessary step a person has to take to avoid gastric acid reflux. In this book, a number of healthy and organic recipes are mentioned that will help a person to enjoy good food and relief in acid reflux conditions as well.

# GERD Diet Cookbook

## Introduction

GERD also called gastric reflux or stomach acid and is a digestive system disorder. It can damage the esophagus, and heartburn is the main symptom of this condition. The esophagus is used for swallowing, and the disease occurs when the acid contained in the stomach returns through the esophagus and inflames it. If you have acid reflux, you may develop a sour or bitter taste in the mouth, and it may cause you to regurgitate food or liquid from the stomach.

One of the causes of GERD is poor nutrition, little variety of diet, little physical activity, lack of sleep, and stress. The best way to treat GERD symptoms is a radical change in lifestyle without smoking and alcohol. Follow a diet and exercise; they can help overcome acid reflux and improve their digestive health.

Studies have shown that between 21 and 40% of people suffer from heartburn. More than 60 million adult Americans suffer from heartburn at least once a month. Although acid reflux occurs in both women and men, men have been shown to have more GERD symptoms.

This book will provide you with many helpful tips on GERD, causes, symptoms, and numerous recipes for getting back to eating without pleasure. That annoying post-meal heartburn. In addition to a healthy diet, we will give particular attention to the correct lifestyle made of sports activities, the importance of sleeping, and reducing stress.

# Chapter 1: Gastro-Esophageal Reflux Disease

Gastroesophageal reflux disease is often caused by reflux into the esophagus of stomach contents and intestinal gases that generate gastroesophageal reflux. This leads to heartburn or throat burning. Occasional small refluxes are considered physiological, for example, once a week, but if the symptom is repeated several times during the week, medical assistance must be requested.

## Causes

GERD is caused due to multiple factors. GERD is caused by numerous factors. It is important to know and identify these reasons and problems. When you are aware of the causes, it is easier to change your lifestyle and improve yourself.

Here are the main causes of GERD:

### Obesity

Obesity is a clinical condition in which the subject has significant accumulations of body fat. This can compromise vital functions and lead to a deterioration in the quality of life. Weight gain can cause problems with bones, body resistance, heart performance, blood circulation, and organ activities. The obese person has an increased abdominal circumference and therefore, an elevated abdominal pressure, which favors the ascent of gastric juices into the esophagus and promotes sphincter incontinence.

### Alcohol

Alcohol is another important cause of GERD. Alcohol is, in fact, already dangerous in itself on people's health. It has been observed that high consumption of alcoholic beverages not only causes acid reflux but increases the risk of a pre-cancerous lesion of the esophagus and the tumor itself.

### Smoke

Smoking is one of the biggest causes of GERD. Smoking affects not only the lungs but also the stomach because nicotine stimulates acid secretion. The combined effect of caffeine and nicotine causes an even higher increase in gastric acidity.

### Low physical activity

As mentioned before, overweight and the consequent increase in the abdominal part is a cause of GERD, so a little physical activity during the week is good for you. You train correctly, with a specific program to your fitness, also following a specific nutritional plan. A healthy diet associated with exercise will be your allies in alleviating symptoms and reducing the probability of complications; your overall health will improve, and your quality of life will definitely have a positive turnaround.

### Diet does not vary

Poor variety in the diet can have a negative effect on your overall health, and GERD can be caused by poor food options. If you consume junk food, snacks, soft drinks, high-fat foods, you may experience acid reflux.

### Bad habits and incorrect posture

GERD can also occur from bad habits such as incorrect posture while eating, such as eating while lying down. Another bad habit is to go to lie on a bed or on the sofa after each meal. It is advisable to take a short walk after eating or at least not to go to bed immediately.

### Pregnancy

GERD is one of the most common ailments in pregnancy because of hormonal changes and the position of the fetus. Usually, this is a problem that mostly affects the past three months.

### Medications

Medications can lead to GERD as a side effect, including nonsteroidal anti-inflammatory drugs, aspirin, and some antibiotics.

## Symptoms

Being aware of the symptoms is essential for healthy living, and starting to understand that we are suffering from GERD. As soon as we feel the symptoms of acid reflux, we must immediately act accordingly to avoid even serious complications. Here are a few major symptoms of gastric acid reflux to consider:

- Heartburn is the most common symptom. It appears as a burning sensation under the chest bone. Pain is caused by irritation of the lining of the esophagus due to the passage of acid that has risen from the stomach.

- Bitter in the back of the mouth and throat

- Burning throat in the upper part

- Even bloody and painful nausea and vomiting in severe cases

- GERD can cause very dark and bleeding stools, accompanied by burning

- Prolonged hiccups accompanied by burning and pain in the throat.

- Feeling that food is stuck in the throat.

- Difficulty in swallowing food, with pain and burning

- Sore throat, a dry cough can occur in the early stages.

- Halitosis and dental erosion are other main symptoms of GERD.

GERD can begin to present itself from the simple burp to the bloody vomit; therefore, one should not take to read these symptoms listed above, even the banalest. It is essential to identify these symptoms initially and to take immediate measures to quickly resolve these problems. Each of the above symptoms does not necessarily address all of them at once, but the symptoms are likely to occur from time to time. So it is important to pay attention to the initial symptoms as well. Sometimes you may have these problems along with other medical conditions, so be sure to discuss them with your doctor first.

## Treatments

GERD is one of the most common digestive disorders involving millions of people around the world. When gastric reflux is not treated properly, it can produce hiatal hernia. It prevents the functioning of the diaphragm regulating valve, which has the task of controlling the flow of food and keeping food in the stomach. You should not underestimate the symptoms in order not to have complications later in your life. It is necessary to chase after treatments. As soon as possible.

Here is some treatment option:

### Lifestyle

Sometimes simply changing your lifestyle is enough to get better in many health conditions. Specifically for GERD, you have to avoid some habits that many people in the world have, including:

- stop smoking
- abuse of alcohol
- Eat quickly by chewing a little
- follow a light diet with few or no spices
- eat small meals and at intervals of time
- lose weight
- avoid chewing gum
- bedtime
- Dress in tight clothes
- Perform substantial physical efforts immediately after meals
- avoid bedtime immediately after eating

### Natural treatments

There are some natural remedies for Gerd that include easily available supplements and herbs. However, they may be useful in combination with what your doctor recommends for GERD

Below is a list of herbs and supplements:

- Ginger root
  is one of the most common natural supplements for stomach problems. It relaxes the muscles in the esophagus and calms the digestive tract. Ginger also improves digestion and consequently helps reduce GERD or reflux because food and acid do not persist in the stomach.

- Licorice root
  calms the stomach. It reduces inflammation of the lining of the esophagus and stomach, which is caused by GERD. It stimulates the body's natural defense mechanisms and is a natural anti-inflammatory.

- Lavender
  its antispasmodic properties it is known to promote proper digestion and to limit the presence of gas in the gastrointestinal level. It is mainly used as an infusion.

- Chicory
  the root can be a very useful digestive aid for people who have GERD. Chicory is also effective for relieving reflux pain because it helps relax the stomach.

- Antioxidants
  antioxidant vitamins A, C, and E are recognized for their potential in preventing GERD. Vitamin supplements are usually used if not enough nutrients are received from food. A blood test can help determine which nutrients your body needs. Your doctor may also prescribe a multivitamin.

- Melatonin
  as the "sleep hormone," melatonin is a hormone produced in the pineal gland. This gland is located in the brain. Melatonin is primarily known for helping initiate sleep.

- Aloe vera
  in reducing the main reflux symptoms

## Medications

- In the early stages of GERD, there are some medications you can use, so remember that you need to consult your doctor before undertaking any drug treatments. With medications, the aim is to reduce esophageal acidity, neutralizing the acid produced, or inhibiting its upstream production. There are different types of medications for gastroesophageal reflux (antacids, histaminergic receptor blockers, proton pump inhibitors) If not in serious cases, it is always to avoid taking them before using them and triggering the vicious circle. It would be good to consider other ways: diet, lifestyle, exercise, reduction of stress, and cigarette smoking. Make sure to consult the physician in severe cases for the medication prescription and regular checkups.

## Risks and complications

If you underestimate the problem and delay with treatments, you can chase complications and risks.

Potential complications of GERD include:

- Esophageal stenosis, which occurs when the esophagus narrows or narrows
- Esophagitis (inflammation of the esophagus)
- Esophageal cancer, which affects a small portion of people with Barrett's esophagus
- Barrett's esophagus, which involves permanent changes to the lining of your esophagus
- Erosion of tooth enamel, gum disease.
- Asthma, chronic cough or other breathing problems

It is essential to solving the problem in the first phase to have adequate and easy-to-perform treatment, thus avoiding reaching more extreme solutions.

# Chapter 2: Prevention from GERD

Yes, prevention is better than cure. You need to make sure you take some essential precautions that will help you live a healthy life. GERD is not caused by external factors such as viruses or infections but only by a wrong daily routine. With a little attention, it is quite easy to follow the prevention guide for GERD related problems.

## Foods to eat and avoid

Most of the problems caused by GERD are related to poor nutrition, so it is necessary to follow a healthy and light diet. Eating correctly is the best method to prevent gastric reflux and allow you to have positive and tangible results in a short period. Now let's see how healthy food can become a valuable ally for prevention, and we will find out what foods to eat and avoid.

### What not to eat

Avoid high-fat foods. These are difficult to digest, and this means they stay in the stomach longer. When foods slow down digestion, the chances of them returning to the esophagus increase, leading to reflux. To avoid this situation, you need to avoid foods such as:

- Animal fat such as lard, bacon, hamburger, pork fat cuts, cold cuts, hot dog, etc
- High-fat snacks that do not have much nutritional value, such as chips, candy, or ice cream.
- Fried foods such as chips, vegetable fries and fried chicken
- salmon, octopus, cuttlefish, mussels, clams, etc.

Protein foods raw or overcooked come:

- Ragout or similar
- Carpaccio, tartare, sushi, etc.
- Braised

Eat less acidic foods:

- Tomato and juice
- Citrus fruits and juice.
- Vinegar

High-calorie foods that can promote overweight:

- Very seasoned foods
- Cheeses
- pasta in an abundant portion

Spices and flavorings
- Chili pepper
- Onion and garlic(In ample quantities)
- Pepper
- All carbonated drinks.

The techniques not recommended are:
- Brazing
- Frying in a pan
- Stewing

## Foods to eat

The following are the foods that must be part of the diet daily to prevent GERD:
- Among the recommended meats there are: chicken, rabbit, turkey, defatted pork or beef muscle, etc
- Among the fishery products: cod, anchovies, sea bream, sea bass, tuna fillet, prawns, etc.
- Among the cheeses: lean ricotta, light spreadable cheese, cottage cheese.
- Among legumes, cereals and derivatives, choose those with medium or low fiber content.
- fruits and vegetables

The recommended cooking techniques are:
- Steam-powered
- In a pressure cooker
- Boil in water
- Baked
- Grilled
- In a pan over low heat.

By following these dietary guidelines, you will take a big step forward to prevent GERD and have a healthy life.

# Impact of Exercise

In the prevention of GERD, physical activity has a significant impact; as it is done after 2/3 hours after the main meal, it will consume all or part of the energy consumed by the food. It will also help you have faster digestion and consequently avoid acid reflux.

## Weight reduction

Overweight or obesity are some of the reasons that can lead to GERD. Regular physical activity will lead to a decrease in weight associated with the correct diet. In general, reducing weight will help you have a better quality of life.

## An active mind and healthy body

An excellent physical activity routine is an excellent combination of body and mind. With daily training, you will consume a lot of your strength and release a lot of the tension you have. With the effort due to a workout, our brain will release the stress hormone, and this will make for a good night's sleep.

## Activate the repair muscles

Exercise and exertion activate the repairing muscles in the body, which help reduce internal and external inflammation. Exercise helps manage this painful condition and enables the body to repair damaged cells.

# Lifestyle changes

To prevent GERD, it is necessary to make changes to your lifestyle, as mentioned in the previous pages. These changes not only help prevent the acid reflux problem but will also give you a better life and avoid further health problems.

## Eat healthily

Healthy eating is the top priority. If you eat fatty foods, refined sugars must be replaced immediately. These foods must be consumed very rarely, only in rare situations. It is necessary to introduce healthy and light food among your food options to avoid such problems.

## Plan your meals

Organizing your meals is essential for the prevention of GERD. Waiting too much between meals is never healthy because it leads to massive meals and consequently, prolonged digestion. It is advisable to make small meals, eat little, and often with meals scheduled with specific intervals that reduce the risk of GERD.

## Do not sleep immediately after a meal

Going to sleep shortly after eating is a bad habit that must be eliminated. The possibility of acid reflux increases as the position taken when sleeping does not guarantee proper digestion.

## Maintain a balance between food options

Changing lifestyles does not mean abandoning all food options. Some foods should be favored over others, but the important thing is knowing how to balance food options and not just eating the same things all the time. Make sure you have many choices in your diet. That will help you have the right food balance.

## Sleep well

Sleep is essential for digestion and stomach food to function well. Sleep is vital to allow digested food and stomach to work well. Make sure you sleep well at least between 7/8 hours. Sleeping little will make you feel tired and will not encourage you to want to exercise.

## Do not stress yourself

Stress and anxiety can affect the proper functioning of the digestive system. Anxiety and stress have effects that fall on the stomach. A stressed brain negatively affects the general function of the organism.

# Chapter 3: Recipes for breakfast

### 1) Maple syrup pancakes

**Ingredients:**
- **Butter 25 g**
- **00 flour 125 g**
- **Medium eggs 2**
- **Fresh whole milk 200 g**
- **Baking powder for cakes 6 g**
- **Brown sugar 15 g**
**TO SEAL:**
**Maple syrup to taste**

We begin the preparation of pancakes by melting the butter on shallow heat, then let it cool. Meanwhile, divide the egg whites from the yolks. Pour the yolks into a bowl and beat them with a hand whisk, then add the melted butter at room temperature and the milk flush, continuing to mix with the whisk. Whisk the mixture until it becomes clear. Add the yeast to the flour and sift everything in the bowl with the egg mixture, mix with the whisk to blend.

Now whip the egg whites that you have kept aside, pouring the sugar little by little, and when they are white and frothy, gently add them to the egg mixture, with movements from top to bottom, to avoid disassembling them. Heat over medium heat (not high; otherwise you will not give the dough time to rise well during cooking, and the pancakes will become too dark) a large non-stick pan (preferably with a thick bottom) and, if necessary, grease with a little butter to spread on the surface with the help of kitchen paper. Pour a ladle of preparation into the center of the saucepan; there will be no need to spread it.

When bubbles begin to appear on the surface, and the base will be golden, turn it on the other side using a spatula, as if it were a crepe or an omelet, then brown the other side in turn, after which the pancake will be ready. Continue with the rest of the dough, and gradually arrange the pancakes on a serving plate, stack them one on top of the other. About 12 pancakes should form with these doses. Serve them hot and sprinkled with maple syrup. You can accompany the pancakes with fresh fruit or sugar of your taste.

### 2) Muffin with chocolate drops

**Ingredients:**
- **Softened butter at room temperature 125 g**
- **00 flour 265 g**
- **Sugar 135 g**
- **Whole milk at room temperature 135 g**
- **Eggs (about 2) at room temperature 110 g**
- **Dark chocolate drops 100 g**
- **Vanilla bean 1**
- **Satin bicarbonate 1 tsp**
- **Salt up to a pinch**
- **Baking powder 1**

To prepare the muffins with chocolate chips worked with the electric whisk butter, left to soften at room temperature for at least an hour previously, with the sugar, until obtaining a frothy and creamy mixture. Then cut a vanilla bean and scrape the seeds using the back of a knife.

Pour the latter into the bowl with butter and sugar. Operate the whips again and add the eggs, also at room temperature, one at a time in this way the ingredients will not untie. Now sift the flour, baking powder, and baking soda directly into the bowl with the mixture.

Also, add a pinch of salt and operate the whisk again to incorporate the powders. You will notice that the dough will become more consistent, then dilute it with milk at room temperature poured flush. At this point, the mixture will be soft and compact.

Add 80 grams of chocolate chips and mix them with a spatula to incorporate them. Then transfer the mixture into a disposable bag without nozzle; in this way, you can do a cleaner job; otherwise, use a spoon as well. Place the paper cups in a muffin pan and fill them 2/3 full, leaving less than an inch from the surface. Each muffin will have to weigh approximately 70 grams.

Pour the remaining 20 drops of chocolate over the cupcakes and bake in a preheated oven at 180 ° for 18-20 minutes in static mode (otherwise at 160 ° for 13-15 minutes if the oven is ventilated). At this point, your chocolate chip muffins are ready to be enjoyed.

### 3) Yoghurt plum cake

**Ingredients:**

- **00 flour 300 g**
- **Eggs (about 5) 300 g**
- **Butter 200 g**
- **Icing sugar 200 g**
- **Low-fat yogurt 150 g**
- **Potato starch 50 g**
- **Baking powder for sweets 15 g**
- **Vanilla bean seeds 1**
- **Salt up to 4 g**

**FOR MOLDS**
- **Butter to taste**
- **00 flour to taste**

To prepare the yogurt plumcake, equip yourself with a mixer equipped with fairly powerful and capacious blades. Place the cubed butter, the seeds of the vanilla bean, the eggs and the flour in the container yogurt, icing sugar, salt, yeast, and starch. Work at maximum speed for about 4 minutes. In the meantime, grease and flour two 16x8 cm slightly flared molds.

As soon as you have obtained a homogeneous mixture, transfer it into the molds. Now dip a blade of a knife, first in the melted butter and then in the center of the two plumcakes. This will ensure uniform growth in cooking. Now put the plumcake in a preheated static oven, and they will have to cook in 2 phases: first at 185 ° for 15 minutes, then at 165 ° for 30 minutes. As soon as they are cooked, take them out of the oven and let them cool completely.

At this point, turn them out and decorate them with icing sugar, and your yogurt plumcakes are ready to taste.

### 4)  Vegetable tart

**Ingredients:**

- **1 pack of puff pastry of about 300 g**
- **2 zucchini**
- **4 potatoes**
- **4 eggs**
- **30 g of grated cheese**
- **basil**
- **chives**
- **extra virgin olive oil**
- **salt**

To make the vegetable tart, start cutting the zucchini. Cut the two ends of the zucchini and cut into slices of about 5mm thick. Salt them slightly and let them drain in a colander. Peel the potatoes, wash and dry them, then cut as if you should make some fried chips by transferring them to a pan in which you have heated two tablespoons of oil.

Brown the potatoes and cook them for 10 minutes. Remove from the heat and put them on paper towels. In the same pan, place the well-dried zucchini and prepare it by turning it often for 15 minutes. In the meantime, beat the eggs. Cook the zucchini, put them in a bowl, add the potatoes and mix everything with the beaten eggs, the grated cheese, the basil, chopped and salted chives.

Brush a tart pan with oil and lay the puff pastry on it. Distribute the filling prepared evenly and bake in a hot oven at 200 ° for about 25 minutes. Then leave the vegetable tart to rest for about ten minutes and serve.

### 5) Potato omelette

**Ingredients:**

- **Eggs 6**
- **Potatoes 500 g**
- **Parmesan cheese 100 g**
- **Parsley to taste**
- **Salt to taste**
- **Seed oil to taste**

To make the potato omelet, first, put some water in a pan and bring to the boil. In the meantime, peel the potatoes and slice them. Now boil the potatoes for about 5 minutes. When cooking the potatoes finely chopped parsley. Now pour the eggs into a bowl, the chopped parsley, the grated cheese, and then salt

At this point, mix to mix the ingredients. Drain the potatoes that have finished cooking, let them cool, and then add them to the egg mixture. Now go to cooking: in a pan heat a drizzle of seed oil, and once it is hot, pour the mixture. Cover with the lid and cook over moderate heat for 15 minutes, turning the pan occasionally. When the surface is not very soft but still damp, turn the omelet over the lid, rotating the pan upside down with a decisive and rapid movement.

Slide the omelet back into the pan to cook the other side, cover again with the lid and continue cooking for another 5 minutes. After this time, the omelet will be ready. You can serve it hot or cold.

## 6) Apple muffin

**Ingredients:**

- **Apples 310 g**
- **00 flour 300 g**
- **Greek yogurt 150 g**
- **Sugar 120 g**
- **Eggs (about 4) 220 g**
- **Baking powder for sweets 16 g**
- **Lemon zest 1**

To make the potato omelet, first, put some water in a pan and bring to the boil. In the meantime, peel the potatoes and slice them. Now boil the potatoes for about 5 minutes. When cooking the potatoes finely chopped parsley. Now pour the eggs into a bowl, the chopped parsley, the grated cheese, and then salt

At this point, mix to mix the ingredients. Drain the potatoes that have finished cooking, let them cool, and then add them to the egg mixture. Now go to cooking: in a pan heat a drizzle of seed oil, and once it is hot, pour the mixture. Cover with the lid and cook over moderate heat for 15 minutes, turning the pan occasionally. When the surface is not very soft but still damp, turn the omelet over the lid, rotating the pan upside down with a decisive and rapid movement.

Slide the omelet back into the pan to cook the other side, cover again with the lid and continue cooking for another 5 minutes. After this time, the omelet will be ready. You can serve it hot or cold.

### 7)  Apple muffin

**Ingredients:**

- **Apples 310 g**
- **00 flour 300 g**
- **Greek yogurt 150 g**
- **Sugar 120 g**
- **Eggs (about 4) 220 g**
- **Baking powder for sweets 16 g**
- **Lemon zest 1**

Start by pouring the eggs into a large bowl and start whipping them with forks or with an electric whisk, then add the sugar little by little continuing to work for about 5 minutes. Add the yogurt and mix it again with the whisk.

Sift the yeast and flour into a separate bowl and add them a spoon at a time, keeping the whisk in action. Finally, add the grated lemon zest and mix again. Now wash the apples, cut them into wedges, and remove the peel. Cut the wedges into cubes and add them to the dough, then mix with a spatula to incorporate them evenly.

Line a muffin pan with paper cups and fill them with about two tablespoons of dough each. Bake in a preheated static oven at 180 ° for about 25-28 minutes. Once cooked, take it out of the oven and let it cool. Your apple muffins are ready to taste!

## 8) Baked Frittata

Ingredients:

- **Eggs 8**
- **Grated cheese 100 g**
- **Chives to taste**
- **Thyme to taste**
- **Salt to taste**
- **Extra virgin olive oil 10 g**

**FOR BRUSHING AND SPREADING THE TRAY**

- **Extra virgin olive oil to taste**
- **Breadcrumbs to taste**

To prepare the frittata, start by oiling a 26x19 cm rectangular baking dish, then line it with breadcrumbs 2. Beat the eggs, add the grated cheese, oil, finely chopped chives. Continue with peeled thyme, salt. Then keep on beating for a few moments until a homogeneous mixture is obtained. Transfer everything to the oven dish and cook in a preheated static oven at 170 ° for 25 minutes. Once ready, serve your frittata in the hot oven to start the day!

## 9) Porridge

Ingredients:

- **Oat flakes 140 g**
- **Whole milk 220 g**
- **Water 200 g**
- **Salt to taste**

**TO SEAL**
- **Honey to taste**

- **Strawberries to taste**
- **Flaked almonds to taste**

To make the porridge first, pour the oats into a bowl, cover with water and leave to soak for about an hour, (it is preferable to leave it to soak the night before). Pour the oats into the saucepan, add the milk, add a pinch of salt and cook the mixture for about 4-5 minutes, stirring often.

When the oats are soft and have absorbed the milk, turn off the heat and transfer the porridge to a bowl and flavor with the honey. Garnish with slices of fresh strawberries and almonds. Serve your lukewarm porridge.

## 10) Salted Plumcake

### Ingredients:

- **00 flour 200 g**
- **Eggs 3**
- **Raw ham 150 g**
- **Whole milk 150 ml**
- **Extra virgin olive oil 60 ml**
- **Salt to taste**
- **Instant yeast for savory preparations 1 sachet**
- **Grated cheese 150 g**

To prepare the salted plumcake, start by sifting the yeast and flour in a bowl, then add the grated cheese. Mix the ingredients well and stir in the raw ham, mix again. Then add the extra virgin olive oil flush. In another bowl, beat the eggs with the milk and salt and add the liquid, thus obtained to the mixture of flour, cheese, and ham.

Stir with a spoon until the ingredients are well mixed. Grease and flour a plumcake mold with a capacity of one liter and put the dough inside. Level it with the back of a spoon and bake in a preheated oven at 180 ° C for 45/50 minutes, doing a toothpick test to check its cooking. When the salted plumcake is cooked, wait until it is warm before removing it from the mold, then let it cool completely. Serve your salted plumcake!

# Chapter 4: Recipes for starter

### 1) Boiled eggs

**Ingredients:**

- **4 fresh eggs**

To prepare the hard-boiled eggs, start by placing the whole eggs in a large saucepan and pour the cold water (the water will have to cover the eggs). Then put the saucepan on the fire and let it boil. From the boil, calculate 9 minutes of cooking. After 9 minutes, remove the saucepan from the heat and pass it under fresh running water to cool the eggs. This will allow you to peel them without getting burned; carefully remove all the shells, then divide the eggs in half, and you will discover the perfectly cooked interior! Boiled eggs are ready to be eaten as you like!

### 2) Cheese waffles

**Ingredients:**

- **Cheese 160 grams**

To prepare the cheese waffles started from the support: cut strips of parchment paper and cut into six squares of about 25 cm, then place a generous spoonful of grated cheese in the center of each.

With the back of the spoon, spread the cheese to form a circle about 20 cm in diameter. Now put each sheet in the oven (also microwave) for a few seconds, at maximum power, until the cheese begins to melt. Cook everything at 180 °, for a few minutes, until the edges of the waffles begin to take on a golden color ( stopping at this step you will have made flat and round waffles; when they have completely cooled, they can already be served).

To give the pods the shape of a "bowl," you have to work them when they are still warm and malleable. It is a rather delicate step because the pods are thin and easily risk breaking. Take a disk of cheese with its parchment paper and place it inside a round or square bowl, then quickly shape it, pressing the cheese towards the bottom with the back of a spoon, until you get the desired shape; then let it cool down.

At this point, you can gently remove the waffles from the bowl, remove the baking paper, and set them aside. Your cheese wafers are ready to be filled with whatever you want.

### 3) Gratinated prawns


**Ingredients:**

- **Gratinated prawns**
- **Shrimp (about 16) 200 g**
- **Salt to taste**
- **White wine 80 ml**

**FOR THE PANURE**
- **Breadcrumbs 50 g**
- **Grana Padano PDO 25 g**
- **Extra virgin olive oil to taste**
- **Parsley to be chopped 10 g**
- **Salt to taste**

We start cleaning the shellfish by peeling them and leaving the tail, cut the back of the shrimp with a knife to eliminate the black thread inside.

Place two prawns in each shell (or in any container of your imagination), to occupy the interior, and pour a spoonful of white wine into each one, directly on the prawns. To prepare the panure: in a bowl, arrange the breadcrumbs, the chopped parsley, the grated Parmigiano, and the salt. Pour a drizzle of oil and mix.

Cover the shells with a few tablespoons of panure and add a drizzle of oil. Arrange the shells with the prawns on a baking tray covered with parchment paper and bake at 180 degrees for about 25 minutes. Now you are ready to serve this imaginative dish!

### 4) Pineapple stuffed with shrimp

**Ingredients:**

- **Pineapple of about 1 kg 1**
- **Shrimp 450 g**
- **Cherry tomatoes 240 g**
- **Chives 6 strands**
- **Mint 5 leaves**
- **Extra virgin olive oil to taste**
- **Salt to taste**
- **Mixed salad**

Let's start by cleaning the prawns (you can also use the frozen ones) by removing the fillet inside. Rinse them under running water, then remove the head with your hands and remove the legs. At this point, shell them. Once all the prawns are cleaned, pour a drizzle of oil into a large pan. Add the peeled prawns in the pan and brown them on both sides. Then turn off the heat and put them in a small bowl to make them cool.

Prepare the pineapple that will be the container for your salad: choose a ripe pineapple and divide it in half. Cut the internal pulp along the perimeter of both halves so as to extract all the pulp without breaking it. Eliminate the most calloused part of the pulp. From the extracted pulp, make medium-sized pineapple cubes to add to the salad. Now chop the aromas: chives and mint.

Then wash the cherry tomatoes under running water, drain, and cut them into small pieces. Take the mixed salad previously washed under water and add the pieces of tomato and also pour the pineapple into pieces. Also, add previously sautéed prawns. Then add the herbs to the salad: chives, minced mint salt, a drizzle of oil, and mix the ingredients to mix the flavors.

Now that the salad is ready, you can start stuffing the pineapple until it is filled. Now you can serve your salad with shrimp in pineapple for a beautiful and fresh summer lunch!

### 5)  Chickpea shrimp and arugula salad

**Ingredients:**

- **Shrimp 1 kg**
- **Pre-cooked chickpeas 240 g**
- **Rocket 150 g**
- **Pine nuts 30 g**
- **TO CONDITION**

- **Lemon juice 1**
- **Balsamic vinegar 1 tsp**
- **Extra virgin olive oil to taste**
- **Salt to taste**

To make the chickpea shrimp and rocket salad, start by cleaning the shrimp (or prawns) by removing the head, the carapace, and the intestines inside. Now toast the pine nuts in a pan for 4-5 minutes until they are browned and set aside. Heat a drizzle of oil in a pan, put the prawns, salt, use a pinch of pepper. Cook them on high heat for 5 -6 minutes. Once cooked, transfer them to a small bowl to cool.

Now drain the pre-cooked chickpeas (you can also use the dried ones but keep them soak and cook them for at least three hours so they will be ready for preparation). In the same pan used for the prawns, heat the chickpeas so that they take on the flavor of the shellfish. Now that all the ingredients are ready, you can compose the salad: In a large bowl, put the washed and dried arugula.

Add the prawns, chickpeas and toasted pine nuts and mix everything together. Finally, take care of the dressing: prepare an emulsion with oil, salt, and the juice of half a lemon. Finish with a teaspoon of balsamic vinegar. Season the salad with the prepared dressing. Your chickpea shrimp and rocket salad are now ready!

### 6)  Vegetable crudités

**Ingredients:**

- **Celery 2**
- **Carrots 2**
- **Fennel 1**
- **Yellow peppers 1/2**
- **1/2 red peppers**
- **Chicory  1**
- **Radishes 12**
- **Extra virgin olive oil to taste**
- **Lemon juice to taste**
- **Salt to taste**

Take two stalks of tender celery and clean them by removing the leaves and any filaments. Cut the stalks into two parts of equal length and then cut the sticks by cutting the pieces obtained for the length. Take the fennel, remove the ends with the leaves, and then also the opposite one; now cut the fennel into four equal parts, which you will reduce again in half.

Take the half peppers, remove the filaments and the internal white parts, then cut the peppers into strips. Remove the radish leaves and wash the radishes under running water.

Peel the carrots, tick the ends, and cut them into parallel slices, which you will then divide into sticks. Remove the outer leaves of the radicchio and keep them fresh and intact by detaching them from its base. Now put the vegetables cut into small glasses and prepare bowls containing extra virgin olive oil. To prepare the sauce, mix together in a salt oil container, lemon, and beat vigorously with a fork to emulsify everything or do it with an immersion blender. Serve your vegetable sticks accompanied by the sauce.

## 7) Chunks of quinoa

### Ingredients:

- **Quinoa 150 g**
- **2 Small zucchini**
- **Eggs 1**
- **Grated cheese 50 g**
- **Grated lemon zest 1**
- **Fresh ginger to be grated to taste**
- **Salt to taste**

Proceed by draining the quinoa and passing it under cold water to stop cooking. At this point, wash the zucchini and peel them, then peel and peel the fresh ginger. Grate the zucchini and place them in a large bowl, where you will add the grated fresh ginger and the grated lemon zest.

Add the boiled quinoa to the grated zucchini, ginger, and lemon zest and add the grated cheese and egg. Season with salt and mix the ingredients until you obtain a homogeneous mixture. Now put the mixture in baking molds (you can also use a non-stick muffin mold) and place them on a baking sheet. Compact the mixture inside the shapes with the help of the back of a spoon, in order to better define the shape of the morsels. Now bake them in an oven already preheated in static mode at 180 ° for 25 minutes (if you use a fan oven cook them at 160 ° for 20 minutes), until the surface is golden brown. At this point, the quinoa morsels are ready to be tasted!

## 8) Eggplant Caviar

**Ingredients:**

- **Round aubergines (about 3) 1 kg**
- **½ lemon juice**
- **Mint 4 leaves**
- **Extra virgin olive oil 2 tbsp**
- **Salt to taste**

Wash the aubergines under running water, then dry them. Arrange them on a dripping pan lined with a sheet of parchment paper. Cook them in a preheated static oven at 180 ° for at least 60 minutes (or at 160 ° for 50 minutes if in a fan oven).

Now remove the aubergines from the oven, and with a knife, remove the peel and with a spoon take the pulp contained inside. Put the pulp in a narrow mesh strainer and with the

back of a spoon press it, so that it releases the excess liquid. Put the pulp in a mixer equipped with blades and add the oil.

Season with salt and add the mint after which operate the blades until you get a thick and homogeneous puree. Transfer everything to a small bowl, then squeeze the juice of half a lemon into the puree you have obtained. Mix everything, and your eggplant caviar is ready to be served.

## 9) Octopus salad

**Ingredients:**

- **Octopus to clean 1 kg**
- **Carrots 1**
- **Celery 1 rib**
- **Laurel 2 leaves**
- **Salt up to 4 g**

**TO CONDITION**
- **Parsley 10 g**
- **Lemon juice 10 g**
- **Extra virgin olive oil 30 g**
- **Black pepper 1 pinch**
- **Salt up to a pinch**

Start with the octopus, rinse it under running water, with a knife cut the bag at eye level to eliminate them, then also remove the beak. Rinse the octopus again under running water and remove the entrails from the bag by washing it carefully inside (You can also use the frozen one). Peel the carrot, then cut it into coarse pieces.

Do the same thing with celery. Place a large saucepan with water on the fire, pour the coast of celery into pieces, the pieces of carrot, the bay leaves, and add the salt. When the water has touched the boil, dip the octopus in the pan and cook over very low heat for 40-45 minutes, covering with a lid. As it cooks, you can remove residues and foam that are created on the surface from the water. At the end of the cooking, let the octopus cool in the same water so that it is soft. Transfer it to the cutting board and, with a knife, separate the head from the tentacles and divide them in half.

Cut the tentacles into small pieces. Cut the head into small pieces and pour everything into a bowl. For the dressing, squeeze the lemon, then wash and finely chop the parsley. Make the dressing by pouring the juice, parsley, lemon juice, oil, and salt into a jar. Close and mix. Pour the mixture over the octopus, mix well, and serve your octopus salad!

## 10) Marinated anchovies

### Ingredients:

- **Anchovies (chopped) 500 g**
- **Lemon juice 150 g**
- **Parsley 20 g**
- **Extra virgin olive oil 140 g**
- **Fine salt**

To prepare the marinated anchovies started with the marinade: pour the parsley together with 40 g of olive oil in a mixer and chop everything for a few moments. Squeeze the lemons, and collect the juice in a container together with the olive oil and season with salt. Mix well and when the two compounds have bonded together, add the chopped parsley.

Keep stirring and keep the marinade aside. Meanwhile, move on to cleaning the anchovies; given that they will not undergo cooking, it is important to make sure that they were cut down during the purchase phase (always choose fresh anchovies to buy in your trusted fish shop); for greater safety, it is recommended to freeze for at least 96 hours at -18 degrees (already gutted) and then thaw to use in the recipe.

 Then take off the head, then pull away the central bone and the entrails, finally rinse the fillets underwater, taking care not to divide the fish into two halves. Place the well-cleaned anchovy fillets side by side in a large container and pour the marinade you have prepared, then cover with plastic wrap. Let stand for at least 5 hours at room temperature.

After the necessary time, remove the film, and finally drain them slightly from the marinade and arrange the marinated anchovies on a plate to serve and enjoy them as an appetizer!

# Chapter 5: First dishes

### 1) Risotto with chickpeas

**Ingredients:**

- **140 grams of brown rice**
- **200 grams of boiled chickpeas**
- **1 carrot**
- **1 teaspoon of extra virgin olive oil**
- **vegetable broth**

Sauté the carrot cut into small pieces with the oil in a pan. Mix and combine 150 grams of boiled chickpeas, giving flavor to everything. Add the rice and continue cooking for 15 minutes or as long as the packaging. Occasionally pour a ladle of vegetable rice broth if you see that the bottom of the pan is dry and without liquid. Cook the rice completely, and at the end of the cooking, add the remaining chickpeas. Your risotto is ready to be eaten!

### 2) Pasta and zucchini

**Ingredients:**

- **Pasta 320 g**
- **Zucchini 650 g**
- **Basil to taste**
- **Salt to taste**
- **Extra virgin olive oil 20 g**
- **Black pepper to taste**
- **Garlic 1 clove**

To prepare pasta and zucchini, boil the water in a large saucepan and salt when it has come to a boil. In the meantime, wash and dry the zucchini, cut them into cubes or slices. In a large enough pan, pour the extra virgin olive oil and heat it over low heat together with a whole clove of garlic already peeled.

As soon as the oil is hot, add the zucchini, add salt and pepper and cook for 5-6 minutes, stirring occasionally, then remove the garlic. In the meantime, boil the pasta in boiling salted water and drain it al dente, keeping some cooking water aside.

Pour the pasta into the pan with the zucchini, together with a little cooking water, sauté the pasta, stir and then turn off. Perfume everything with a little chopped basil by hand, and your pasta and zucchini are ready to be enjoyed.

### 3) Legumes and cereals soup

**Ingredients:**

- **Mixed legumes + cereals 500 g**
- **Carrots 2**
- **2 ribs celery**
- **Onions 1**
- **Medium potatoes 2**
- **Auburn tomatoes 200 g**
- **Grana Padano DOP crusts 2**
- **Garlic 1 clove**
- **Vegetable broth 1 l**
- **Extra virgin olive oil 3 tbsp**
- **1 sprig rosemary**
- **Thyme 1 sprig**
- **Bay leaf 1 leaf**
- **Sage 1 sprig**

Soak the cereals in cold water the day before. The following day drain them well, then prepare a mixture with onion, garlic, celery, and carrots. Fry the mince in the oil in a large pot or in a crock, then add the drained cereals and legumes, mix for a minute, and then cover with the vegetable broth. Add the tomatoes, previously peeled and cut into cubes. Grate the Grana Padano crusts and add them to the pan.

At this point, add the bunch of aromatic herbs, which you can stop by tying it to the handle of the pot so that they do not scatter in the soup, and you can easily eliminate once cooked. Slowly bring the soup to a boil, add salt and then cover the pan with a lid, cook slowly for at least an hour, adding, if necessary, more vegetable broth so that the soup remains with the right amount of liquid. Half an hour before the end of cooking, add the peeled and diced potatoes. When cooked, remove the aromatic bunch, add a drizzle of extra virgin olive oil and serve in bowls or holsters.

### 4) Lentil soup

**Ingredients:**
- **Lentils 250 g**
- **2 ribs celery**
- **Carrots 2**
- **White onions 1**
- **Small potatoes 2**
- **2 cloves garlic**
- **Zucchini 2**
- **Laurel 2 leaves**
- **Cumin 1 tsp**
- **Cloves 2**
- **Extra virgin olive oil 2 tbsp**
- **Salt to taste**
- **Boiling water 2,5 l**

Soak the lentils in cold water the day before. After the soaking time, start cleaning the vegetables, and finely cut the carrots, after peeling them, the celery (without the leaves), the zucchini and the potatoes.

Heat the oil with the garlic in a saucepan with high sides; finely chop the onion and add it to the pan; stew it gently and then add all the vegetables except the lentils. Cook on low heat for about 10 minutes, stirring with a wooden spoon; when they are softened, add the lentils well drained from the soaking water, the bay leaves and the cloves, also pour the cumin powder and add the salt; lastly, pour the hot water, or vegetable broth, bring gently to a boil, cover with a lid and cook over low heat for about 2 hours, or until the lentils are well cooked and tender (but not unmade); if necessary, add more water if the soup dries out too much.

Before bringing to the table, remove the bay leaves and possibly also the cloves and serve hot.

### 5) Quinoa with vegetables

#### Ingredients:

- **Quinoa 200 g**
- **Champignon mushrooms 100 g**
- **Red peppers 70 g**
- **Yellow peppers 70 g**
- **Zucchini 150 g**
- **Red onions 100 g**
- **Water 400 g**
- **Extra virgin olive oil to taste**
- **Mint to taste**
- **Salt to taste**
- **Black pepper to taste**

To prepare the quinoa with vegetables, start by cleaning the red onions and cutting them finely. Cut the red pepper in half and remove the internal seeds. Then cut it into cubes and repeat the same thing also for the yellow pepper. Cut the zucchini into cubes, and finally clean the mushrooms and cut them into slices.

Heat the oil in a pan and add the onions. Let them stew slowly, blending with a little water when they begin to brown, and continue cooking for a few minutes until they are very tender. Once this is done, add the peppers, mix, and cook a couple of minutes before adding zucchini and mushrooms. Cook five more minutes, adding salt and pepper. Your vegetables are ready and beautiful crispy! Now take care of the quinoa: rinse it thoroughly, then heat oil on the bottom of a pan and pour the quinoa to toast it.

Stir with a wooden spoon to prevent it from sticking to the bottom and add the salt. Continue to cook and cover with the rest of the water: its volume must be twice that of quinoa. As soon as the seeds open to flower and the water has been absorbed, the quinoa is ready, and at that point, you can combine them with the vegetables. Mix and skip a minute to tie the flavors, then add with a handful of mint leaves. The quinoa with vegetables is ready to be enjoyed!

### 6)  Spaghetti with tuna

**Ingredients:**

- **Spaghetti 320 g**
- **Tuna in oil (drained) 150 g**
- **Peeled tomatoes 400 g**
- **Extra virgin olive oil to taste**
- **Salt to taste**
- **Black pepper to taste**
- **Basil to taste**
- **Golden onions ½**

To prepare the spaghetti with tuna, start by heating the water in a saucepan and add salt to the boil, cook the pasta. In the meantime, drain the tuna fillet from the conservation oil. Clean the onion and slice it thinly. Olive oil in a pan and add the chopped onion. Let it dry on the heat for a few minutes, stirring often.

 Remove the tuna with your hands and add it to the pan when the onion has dried and let it brown for a couple of minutes, stirring constantly. Now, mash the peeled tomatoes with a fork and pour them into the pan with the tuna, let the sauce cook for about 10 minutes.

In the cooking time of the seasoning, also the pasta will be ready. Drain the spaghetti directly into the pan with the tuna, season with ground pepper, turn off the heat, and season with fresh basil leaves. Stir and serve your hot tuna spaghetti!

### 7) Chickpea and pumpkin soup

### Ingredients:

- **Delica pumpkin to clean 600 g**
- **Drained pre-cooked chickpeas 400 g**
- **Beets 100 g**
- **Golden onions 100 g**
- **Juniper berries 3 berries**
- **Laurel 2 leaves**
- **Water 1.5 l**
- **Extra virgin olive oil to taste**
- **Salt to taste**
- **Black pepper to taste**

To make the chickpea and pumpkin soup, first of all, clean the onion and slice it finely. Now clean the pumpkin: cut it in half, then empty it of the seeds internally and remove the peel: in all, you will need 430 g of clean pumpkin. Cut the pulp until diced. Wash the beets and cut them into thin strips.

Pour the olive oil into a pan, then add the sliced onion and the juniper berries. Leave to cook over low heat until the onion is soft. At this point, add the pumpkin, brown it over medium heat and then wet with a little water taken from the total dose. Add the chickpeas, and the chard reduced to 11 strips, salt, pepper, and the rest of the water necessary for cooking.

Flavored with bay leaves, stir, cover with a lid and cook over high heat for 15 minutes. Remove the lid and continue to cook for another 15 minutes. Remove the bay leaves and juniper berries and serve your soup with a drizzle of raw oil and minced black pepper. The pumpkin and chickpea soup are ready to be served.

### 8) Pasta with eggplants

**Ingredients:**

- **Striped Sedanini 320 g**
- **Aubergines 350 g**
- **Cherry tomatoes 250 g**
- **Basil a few leaves**
- **Fresh spring onion 100 g**
- **Salt to taste**
- **Black pepper to taste**
- **Extra virgin olive oil 30 g**

To prepare the pasta with the aubergines washed and then diced around the aubergines. Then transfer them to a colander, salt them lightly and place a saucer with a weight on top of them and let them drain for a couple of hours. When the aubergines have removed all the water, start cutting the spring onion into thin slices. Pour the oil into a pan, let it warm up, and add the spring onion. Once it is golden brown, add the aubergines, salt, pepper, and cook for about 15 minutes. Now wash the tomatoes and cut them into wedges and add them to the aubergines only when they are tender and cooked.

Season with salt and pepper and cook for another 4-5 minutes. In the meantime, cook the pasta in abundant boiling salted water. Once al dente, drain it and pour it directly into the pan with the aubergines. Skip your pasta with the aubergines by adding the basil leaves 1, now you just have to bring to the table.

## 9) Vegetable pie

### Ingredients:

- **Aubergines 80 g**
- **Zucchini 160 g**
- **Red potatoes 190 g**
- **Peppers 300 g**
- **Smoked scamorza 260 g**
- **PDO Parmesan Cheese 100 g**
- **Breadcrumbs 120 g**
- **Salt to taste**
- **Extra virgin olive oil to taste**

**FOR THE TRAY**
- **Butter to taste**
- **Breadcrumbs to taste**

To prepare the vegetable pie, start by washing and drying all the vegetables. Prepare the aubergines and peel them and divide them in half and then make slices about 1cm thick (you can help yourself with a mandolin).

Do the same with the zucchini and finally slice the potatoes without removing the peel. Now take the peppers and remove them from the top, divide them in half and then remove the seeds and filaments. Finally, divide into six parts. Finally, slice the scamorza of the same thickness as the vegetables. Grease a baking dish and line the base with the breadcrumbs.

Now move on to composing the layers. Start with the aubergine slices by placing them all on the base. Sprinkle with oil, salt; then add a few slices of scamorza cheese, a little parmesan, and breadcrumbs. Then arrange the slices of zucchini, sprinkle with salt and oil, then distribute the scamorza, parmesan, and breadcrumbs. Finally, again with peppers.

Season with salt, oil, parmesan, the breadcrumbs, and start again with the last layer: the potato layer. On the last layer sprinkle with oil and finish with salt, parmesan, and breadcrumbs. Then proceed with the cooking in a static oven, preheated to 180 °, for about 70 minutes 20. Once ready, let it cool. Transfer to a serving dish.

## 10) Rice cake
### Ingredients:

- **Champignon mushrooms 500 g**
- **Rice 300 g**
- **Grated cheese 150 g**
- **½ white onions**
- **Vegetable broth about 750 ml**
- **White wine 60 ml**
- **Parsley 1 sprig**
- **Salt to taste**

To prepare the rice cake, start cleaning and chopping the onion. Then dedicate yourself to the champignon mushrooms, wash and clean them, then remove the part of the stem with the roots and cut the head of the champignons into rather thin slices.

 Chop the fresh parsley. In a large pan, pour a drizzle of oil then add the champignon mushrooms and the chopped parsley. Fry over low heat for about 3 minutes, then add 30ml of white wine. Stir and cook the mushrooms for about 5 minutes. Season with salt and then cook for about 10 minutes on moderate heat. The mushrooms will not have to cook completely because then they will complete cooking in the oven.

While the mushrooms are cooking, pour the oil into a large pan, add the previously chopped onion and leave to fry for about 5 minutes. Then pour the rice, sauté for a couple of minutes mixing with a wooden spoon and pour the remaining ml of white wine. Continue cooking the risotto for about 20 minutes, adding the vegetable broth with a ladle little by little when you see that the rice is free of liquid.

When there are 2 minutes left to cook the rice, pour the grated cheese, stir, turn off the heat and let the risotto rest for a few minutes. Take a baking sheet and cover it with parchment paper. Then with a spoon, start to create a layer of rice, compacting it with the back of the spoon.

When you have covered the bottom, create a layer of mushrooms, then rice, so that the result is two layers with the mushroom filling. Finally, sprinkle the surface with the leftover cheese. Finally, bake in a preheated static oven at 200 ° for about 30 minutes (if oven at 180 ° for about 25 minutes). Then take it out of the oven and let it cool down.

# Chapter 6: Main courses

### 1) Veal roast, apples and potatoes

Ingredients:

- 600 grams of veal fillet
- 1 teaspoon of oil
- 2 sprigs of rosemary
- half a glass of white wine
- 2 apples
- 250 grams of potatoes
- Salt

Put the meat in a pan with oil, rosemary, and a pinch of salt. Brown it by blending with the white wine. Combine the apples with the peel and the chopped potatoes. Bake at 200 degrees for about 30 minutes. Get out of the oven, remove the meat, and let it cool. Cut it into slices and serve with potatoes and apples.

### 2) Poached eggs

Ingredients:

- Very fresh, organic eggs 4
- Coarse salt to taste
- White wine vinegar 10 g
- TO ACCOMPANY
- 4 slices bread

When the salt has dissolved, and the water starts to boil lightly (it must not boil strongly), lower the flame and with a whisk stir always in the same direction to create a vortex in the water; then break an egg into a small bowl and pour it in the center of the vortex. Cook the egg like this for 2 minutes. Do not mix or move the egg. Drain the egg with the help of a slotted spoon, then lay it on the toasted bread and serve your hot poached eggs.

### 3) Prawns stewed

Ingredients:

- King prawns (12 pieces) 600 g
- Peeled tomatoes (cherry tomatoes) 400 g
- Water 200 g
- Brandy 50 g
- Extra virgin olive oil 30 g
- Garlic 1 clove
- Parsley to taste
- Salt to taste

To prepare the prawns stewed, start cleaning the prawns: remove only the carapace that surrounds them and remove the dark filament, gently pulling it with the blade of the knife or a toothpick. Leave the head and tail attached and lay the prawns on a tray. In a pan, heat the olive oil, then add a whole peeled garlic clove. When the oil is hot, place the prawns in a pan, one next to the other without overlapping them, brown them on both sides for 1 minute, then blend with the brandy, then add the peeled cherry tomatoes and stretch the sauce with water.

Salt and cover with the lid and continue cooking for about 5 minutes. Remove the garlic clove with kitchen tongs, then mash a portion of the cherry tomatoes with a fork and continue cooking the prawns for about 10 minutes. Wash, dry and finely chop the parsley. When cooked, turn off the heat and flavor the prawns with fresh parsley and serve them on the table hot.

### 4)   Sea bass with herb in salt crust

Ingredients:

- Salt up to 1 kg
- Sea bass (sea bass) 800 g
- Coarse salt 1 kg
- Sage 6 leaves
- Thyme 6 sprigs
- Parsley 1 bunch
- Dill 2 tufts
- Laurel 4 leaves
- Rosemary 3 sprigs
- Egg whites about 4
- Garlic 1 clove
- Lemons 1

Spread a sheet of parchment paper on a baking sheet and then lay a thin layer (about 1.5 cm) of the mixture obtained, which will form the cooking bed for the sea bass. Now place the sea bass on the bed of salt that you previously flavored by placing it in your belly

aromatic herbs, minced garlic, and lemon zest; now cover the sea bass with the salt mixture by pressing it gently to make the dough adhere well and give a shape that adheres to the fish 11. Bake for about 40 minutes (if instead of 1-kilo sea bass, you have taken a smaller one 400 / About 500gr the cooking time will be about 25-30 minutes). After 40 minutes, remove the sea bass from the oven, let it rest for a few moments, then, using a small hammer, break the salt crust and proceed to remove the skin of the fish. Open it in two by removing the central bone, as in any other oven preparation. You can accompany the sea bass, with boiled potatoes, or also cooked in the oven. Season with a drizzle of extra virgin olive oil, not to cover the aroma and delicate flavor of the sea bass.

## 5) Chicken and zucchini salad

Ingredients:

- Sliced chicken breast 400 g
- Zucchini 200 g
- Eggplants 200 g
- Datterini tomatoes 150 g
- Mixed salad 60 g
- Salt to taste
- Extra virgin olive oil to taste
- 

**FOR MARINATING**

- Extra virgin olive oil 25 g
- Wildflower honey 25 g
- ½ lemon juice
- Thyme to taste
- Salt to taste

To prepare the chicken and zucchini salad, we must first marinate the chicken. Arrange the chicken breasts in an ovenproof dish, pour the oil inside, season with salt, the juice of half a lemon, honey, and a few sprigs of thyme. Turn the slices over both so that the entire surface of the meat is well marinated, then cover the baking dish with plastic wrap and let it sit for one hour at room temperature.

Now move on to the preparation of the vegetables. Wash the zucchini, cut the ends, and cut them lengthwise with a sliced knife about 1 cm thick. Do the same thing with eggplants too. Finally, wash and cut the cherry tomatoes into pieces. Now heat the grill, grease it with a drizzle of oil, then lay the slices of zucchini and grill them on both sides, then salt.

Also, grill and salt the aubergines, turning them on both sides, then switch to the chicken, which you will pick from the marinade to put it on the grill. Once grilled, cut the aubergines, zucchini, and chicken slices into strips about 2 cm long.

Let the grilled vegetables cool, then transfer them to a bowl, add the cherry tomatoes, the chicken and the mixed salad, previously washed and dried, then mix and transfer to the dishes. The chicken and zucchini salad are ready to be served!

### 6)  Pan-fried sea bream

**Ingredients:**

- **Sea bream (2 pieces) 1100 g**
- **Extra virgin olive oil 30 g**
- **Carrots 150 g**
- **Courgettes 150 g**
- **Fresh spring onion 70 g**
- **Garlic 1 clove**
- **Thyme to taste**

To prepare the sea bream in a pan, first of all, you have to clean the fish (otherwise you can buy it already gutted). Make a cut on the belly with scissors and remove the entrails with your hands, then rinse the inside thoroughly under water and eliminate the scales using a blade of a knife; do this under running water so as not to spread the scales around.

Now let's cut the vegetables: wash and peel the carrots, then cut the ends and cut them into rounds. Wash and peel the courgettes and cut them into cubes.

Finally, wash the onion, remove the base, and cut it into rounds. Pour the oil into a large non-stick pan, add a clove of poached garlic and fry it for a couple of minutes. When the oil is flavored, remove the garlic from the pan and lay the sea bream inside, then add the zucchini, carrots, spring onion, and thyme sprigs and salt to taste.

Cover the pan with a lid and cook over medium heat for 7 minutes, then turn the sea bream with the help of 2 spatulas being careful not to break them; cover again with the lid and cook for another 7 minutes. Cooking times may vary depending on the weight of the sea bream you will use. Pan-fried sea bream is ready to eat!

### 7)   Cod medallions and broccoli

Ingredients:

- **Cod fillet 400 g**
- **Broccoli 200 g**
- **Potatoes 400 g**
- **Marjoram 3 sprigs**
- **Extra virgin olive oil to taste**
- **Salt to taste**

- **TO ACCOMPANY**
- **Cherry tomatoes 200 g**
- **Dried oregano to taste**
- **Extra virgin olive oil to taste**
- **Salt to taste**

To prepare the medallions of cod and broccoli, first, we take the cod fillets (they should also be frozen well, in that case, let them thaw for at least 2-3 hours before). Then put two saucepans on the fire with water to bring to a boil; in one dip the potatoes, calculate them 30-40 minutes. The time may vary depending on the size of the potatoes, so remember to check the degree of cooking with a fork.

If the fork easily penetrates inside the potatoes, it means it is cooked. In the meantime, wash the broccoli, put them in the other pan, and when the water boils boil them for about 5 minutes. After 5 minutes, drain the broccoli and coarsely chop them, then let them cool. When the potatoes are ready, peel and mash them with a potato masher in a large bowl, then preheat the oven to 200 ° in static mode.

Finally, take the cod fillets and cut them into several, not too small parts. When the vegetables have cooled, take the bowl where you have mashed the potatoes, add the chopped broccoli and cod, salt and add the marjoram leaves, then knead with your hands to mix all the ingredients. Take some dough and shape it with a pastry cutter to form the medallions.

Place the medallions on a dripping pan lined with parchment paper, season with a little oil, then cook in a preheated static oven at 200 ° for about 20 minutes. While the medallions are in the oven, move on to the preparation of the side dish: wash and cut the cherry tomatoes in half; heat the oil in a pan and put the cherry tomatoes, add the salt and oregano and cook over medium heat for about 15 minutes.

After the cooking time of the medallions, take them out of the oven and transfer them to a serving dish; lay the still hot tomatoes on one side, add a few leaves of marjoram and season with a drizzle of raw oil. Your cod and broccoli medallions are ready to be brought to the table!

### 8) Baked chicken legs

**Ingredients:**

- **Chicken legs 4**
- **Potatoes 500 g**
- **Salt to taste**
- **Extra virgin olive oil 50 g**
- **Rosemary 3 sprigs**
- **Thyme 3 sprigs**

Put the chicken legs in a baking dish and season with salt, oil, and marinate. Peel the potatoes, cut them into wedges, and transfer them into a dripping pan lined with parchment paper. Season with salt, oil (optional pepper but do not overdo it), then add the chicken legs and flavor everything with the sprigs of thyme and rosemary. Bake in a preheated static oven at 180 ° for 80 minutes, turning them halfway through cooking. When they are golden brown, take them out of the oven and serve them!

### 9) Stuffed potatoes

#### Ingredients:

- **Potatoes (4 of the same size) 860 g**
- **Ground beef 120 g**
- **Sweet provola 40 g**
- **Grated Parmesan cheese 40 g**
- **Extra virgin olive oil 30 g**
- **White wine 15 g**
- **Salt to taste**

To prepare the baked stuffed potatoes, start by washing and drying the potatoes well. It is advisable to choose potatoes of the same size in order to obtain uniform cooking afterward. Arrange the potatoes on a dripping pan covered with parchment paper. Cook them in a static preheated oven at 190 ° C for about  1 hour (the cooking times depend on the size of the potatoes, to regulate your cooking, test them by skewering the potatoes with a toothpick).

In the meantime, heat the oil in a pan and add the minced meat. Crush it to crumble and brown it for about 10 minutes, then blend with white wine, and once the alcohol has evaporated, turn off the heat and keep aside. When the potatoes have finished cooking, take them out of the oven, let them cool, then divide them in half lengthwise. With a teaspoon, take the pulp of the potato, leaving a border of about half a centimeter and collect it in a bowl.

Once you have dug out the potatoes, mash the pulp to obtain a puree, add the browned and salted mince. Cut the provola into cubes, add it to the mixture, mix, and mix the ingredients well. Now stuff your potatoes with the filling.

Season the potatoes with the grated cheese, then lay them on a dripping pan covered with parchment paper and bake at 180 ° C for 5 minutes to brown the surface. Serve your stuffed baked potatoes hot.

### 10) Roasted rabbit

**Ingredients:**

- **Rabbit in pieces 1.2 kg**
- **4 sprigs rosemary**
- **Salt to taste**
- **Vegetable broth 150 g**
- **Potatoes 800 g**
- **Red onions 120 g**
- **Thyme 4 sprigs**
- **White wine 40 g**
- **Bay leaf 1 leaf**
- **Extra virgin olive oil 70 g**

To prepare the rabbit in the oven, start by preparing the vegetable broth a couple of hours before, chop the rosemary, then transfer half of it into a pan where you have poured 40 g of oil.

Add a bay leaf and leave to flavor over low heat for 2-3 minutes. At this point, raise the heat and add the pieces of rabbit, let them brown on both sides for 3-4 minutes, salt and blend with the white wine. Once the alcoholic phase has evaporated, add a ladle of broth, and cook over low heat for another 5-6 minutes.

Meanwhile, prepare the potatoes, peel them, and cut them into fairly large pieces. Also, cut the onion and transfer everything to a bowl, flavored with chopped rosemary and kept aside previously, the thyme leaves, salt.

Sprinkle with 20 g of oil and mix potatoes and onions to flavor them.

Transfer everything to a large pan, oiled with about 10 g of oil. Then also arrange the browned pieces of rabbit.

Add the remaining vegetable broth and cook the rabbit together with the potatoes in a static oven preheated to 200 ° for 40 minutes. Once baked, serve your rabbit in the oven!

# Chapter 7: Recipes for Side dish

### 1)  Fennel in a pan

**Ingredients:**

- **Fennel (about 2) 900 g**
- **Extra virgin olive oil 15 g**
- **Himalayan salt (pink) to taste**
- **Marjoram to taste**
- **Thyme to taste**

To make the fennel in a pan, start by washing the fennel, then clean them by cutting the base of the core, and the stalks, after which cut them into wedges.

Once the fennel is cut, you can proceed with cooking: heat the extra virgin olive oil in a pan, then add the fennel wedges and cook for about 5 minutes on high heat. Season with the Himalayan salt and season with the leaves of marjoram and thyme. Continue cooking for another 5 minutes to keep the fennel crunchy otherwise, and you can continue cooking them for a few more minutes if you like them softer. Serve your fennel hot in a pan.

### 2)  Baked aubergines

**Ingredients:**

- **2 cloves garlic**
- **Extra virgin olive oil to taste**
- **Salt to taste**
- **Aubergines 970 g**
- **Auburn tomatoes 500 g**
- **Chopped parsley 3 tbsp**

To prepare the baked aubergines, you can use both the rotunda and the elongated violet variety. First, wash the aubergines and cut them into slices. Salt the aubergine slices and place them in a colander. Cover them with a plate on which you will put weight in order to compress them and leave them for half an hour so that they lose the bitter liquid. Meanwhile, wash the tomatoes, cut them in half, and dig the inside gently with a small knife to remove the seeds. Now cut them into small pieces and pour them into a bowl.

Now season the tomatoes: add the garlic cloves and the three spoons of finely chopped parsley, the oil, and the salt. Mix and let the pieces of tomatoes macerate with the dressing for a few minutes. Meanwhile, after half an hour, pick up the slices of eggplant and check that they have released the bitter water. Rinse them under running cold water and then dry them with kitchen paper or cloth. Heat the static oven to 180 ° -200 °. Grease a high-sided baking pan with olive oil and start forming a layer of aubergines.

Then cover with a layer of cherry tomatoes. Continue in this way until you have used up all the aubergines. Then bake the dish in a preheated static oven and cook at 200 ° for at least 40 minutes. You can eat both hot and cold.

### 3) Grilled vegetables

**Ingredients:**

- **Courgettes 300 g**
- **Eggplants 450 g**
- **Peppers 850 g**
- **Tomatoes 200 g**
- **Salt to taste**

To prepare the grilled vegetables, wash all the vegetables under running fresh water, and dry them. Cut the zucchini and aubergines into slices; take the peppers, remove the upper part, divide them in half, and with a knife remove the white filaments and the seeds that are inside. Cut them into rather large cubes and set aside. Remove the stalk of the tomatoes and cut them into rounds. Cut all the vegetables, heat the grill.

When the grill is hot, cook the vegetables a little at a time. Spread the peppers close to each other, grilling them for 5 minutes and turning them over for even cooking, then put the eggplants on the fire for 3 minutes and continue with the courgettes for another 3 minutes. Remember to always turn the vegetables over for even cooking.

Finish with the tomatoes cooking for 4 minutes until they are well grilled. Finally, season the grilled vegetables with olive oil and salt.

### 4) Mashed potatoes

**Ingredients:**

- **Yellow floury potatoes 1 kg**
- **Whole milk 200 g**
- **Butter 30 g**
- **Parmesan cheese to be grated 30 g**
- **Salt to taste**
- **Nutmeg to taste**

Let's start by boiling the potatoes. Then pour them in a large pot and cover with plenty of water. Put the pan on the fire, and when the water has boiled, it will take 40 to 50 minutes. The cooking times depend on the size of the potatoes. Reached the 40 minutes of cooking skewer a potato with a fork and see if it penetrates easily; at that point, it is cooked. Drain and let it cool for a few minutes because you will have to take advantage that the potatoes are still very hot to peel them easily.

After peeling the potatoes, pour them into the potato masher, pour them directly into the cooking pan. Then add a pinch of salt and flavor by grating a little nutmeg. In the meantime, put the milk in a saucepan.

Meanwhile, light over a low flame where there is a pot with the mashed potatoes, and when the milk is hot, pour it inside and mix with a whisk until the mixture is well blended. Then turn off the heat and stir adding butter and Parmesan cheese. Your mashed potato is read.

### 5) Baked au gratin vegetables

**Ingredients:**

- **Zucchini 300 g**
- **Aubergines 180 g long**
- **Red peppers 250 g**
- **Yellow peppers 250 g**
- **Extra virgin olive oil 20 g**
- **Salt to taste**

**FOR BREADING**

- **Breadcrumbs 30 g**
- **Parmesan cheese DOP to be grated 30 g**
- **Dried oregano to taste**

First, cut the vegetables: wash the aubergines, remove the ends, and cut them diagonally into slices 2-3 cm thick; do the same thing with the zucchini. Finally, wash the peppers, empty them of the seeds and internal filaments and cut them first in half and then into pieces more or less as big as the slices of aubergines and zucchini.

Arrange the cut vegetables in a pan lined with parchment paper, then season with salt and olive oil 6. Bake the pan in a static preheated oven at 180 ° for 45 minutes. In the meantime, prepare the breadcrumbs for the vegetables: In a bowl, add the breadcrumbs with the grated Parmesan and the oregano, and mix well.

After 45 minutes, remove the vegetables from the oven, spread the breadcrumbs over all the vegetables with a spoon. Bake at 180 ° again for another 15 minutes. Your side dish is ready!

### 6) Artichoke salad

Ingerdients:

- **Artichokes (about 6) 1 kg**
- **1 Lemons for acidulated water**

**FOR THE CITRONETTE**

- **Lemon juice 30 g**
- **Salt to taste**
- **Black pepper to taste**
- **Extra virgin olive oil 60**

Start by cleaning the artichokes: prepare the acidulated water to store the artichokes without oxidizing them as you clean them. Fill a bowl with water and squeeze the juice of 1 lemon inside. Remove part of the stem of the artichokes and the more leathery leaves. With a knife cut off the tip and the outermost part of the stem to keep the inside tender. Clean the artichoke, divide it into two equal parts, thinly slice the artichokes, and place them in the bowl with acidified water as you cut them. Once the cleaning is finished, put them to drain in a colander. In the meantime, take care of the seasoning.

Squeeze 30 g of lemon juice and add it to 60 g of olive oil, salt and mix the emulsion with a whisk. Pour the artichokes into a bowl and flavor them with the citronette, mix and then serve the salad on the serving dishes!

### 7) Breadcumb Potatoes

Ingredients:

- **Potatoes 1 kg**
- **2 sprigs rosemary**
- **Bread crumbs 50 g**
- **Breadcrumbs 20 g**
- **Sage 3 leaves**

- **Extra virgin olive oil to taste**
- **Salt to taste**

Peel the potatoes and cut them into wedges, then place them in a bowl with water so as not to blacken them. Meanwhile, finely chop the sage, rosemary, and set aside. Now take the breadcrumbs and add the breadcrumbs and the chopped herbs. Now drain the potato wedges with a strainer and pour the chopped breadcrumbs and season with a drizzle of olive oil and salt.

Stir and pour into a baking tray lined with parchment paper and cover the potatoes with a spoonful of breadcrumbs. Bake the potatoes in a static oven at 180 ° for 40 minutes (if the oven is at 160 ° for 30 minutes). When cooked, your potatoes will be golden and crispy, take them out of the oven and let them cool before serving.

## 8) Crunchy salad

**Ingredients:**

- **Iceberg salad 1 large head**
- **PDO Parmigiano Reggiano one piece or in flakes 80 g**
- **Carrots 2**
- **4 slices sandwich bread**
- **Chopped parsley 3 tbsp**
- **Anchovies fillets 8**
- **Lemon juice**
- **Salt to taste**
- **Extra virgin olive oil 2 tablespoons for frying, plus q.s. to season**

Wash the iceberg salad leaves, cut them finely, and put them in a large salad bowl. Now pass the carrots and with a potato peeler cut the carrots finely with a potato peeler; always with the potato peeler, do the same also with the Parmesan cheese.

Chop the anchovy fillets and parsley and place them in a bowl with oil, salt and mix everything with a fork and leave them for a few minutes to rest. Take the slices of sandwich bread, remove the darker edges, and cut them into 1 cm cubes on each side.

In a pan, add two tablespoons of extra virgin olive oil, heat it and then throw it into the cubes of bread over moderate heat, turning them on all sides. Once golden, place them on absorbent kitchen paper 11. Add the carrots, Parmesan, and the oil and parsley dressing to the iceberg salad. Mix the ingredients and then add the crispy croutons 15. Ready-made salad!

### 9)  Ginger gourd

**Ingredients:**

- **Pumpkin 1 kg**
- **Fresh ginger 40 g**
- **Leeks 1**
- **Vegetable broth 500 ml**
- **Extra virgin olive oil 20 g**
- **Salt to taste**

Let's start by cleaning the pumpkin, cut it in half, empty it of the seeds and internal filaments, remove the peel, and cut it into cubes. And cut it into small cubes. Wash the leek, peel it and keep the white part of the stem that you will slice in thin slices. Place a large pan on the heat, pour the leeks and season with the olive oil and fry until the leek is wilted (about 5 minutes).

At this point, pour a ladle of hot broth and add the ginger and the pumpkin cubes and salt. Pour another ladle of broth and cook over medium heat for about 25-30 minutes, adding broth little by little during cooking so as not to dry the vegetables too much. When the pumpkin is soft, turn off the heat.

The ginger pumpkin is ready to be brought to the table.

### 10) Roasted carrots with pistachio

**Ingredients:**

- **Carrots 650 g**
- **Unsalted pistachios 80 g**
- **Rosemary 3 sprigs**
- **Salt to taste**
- **Extra virgin olive oil to taste**

Wash the carrots, peel them, divide them in half and then make some sticks by cutting them for the long side. Pour the carrots into a bowl and season with rosemary, olive oil, and salt. Now roughly chop the pistachios with a knife.

Add the pistachios to the carrots and mix them to amalgamate all the ingredients. Line a baking sheet with parchment paper and pour the carrots trying to distribute them evenly in order to facilitate cooking. Bake in a preheated static oven at 220 ° for 30 minutes. Once cooked, take the roasted carrots out of the oven and let them cool before serving.

# Chapter 8: Recipes for dessert

### 1) Cake Seven Jars

### Ingredients:

- **Natural white yogurt (125 ml) at room temperature 1 jar**
- **Brown sugar 2 jars**
- **00 flour 2 jars**
- **Potato starch 1 jar**
- **Seed oil 1 jar**
- **Baking powder for sweets 16 g**
- **Medium eggs at room temperature 3**

To prepare the cake seven jars, take a 125 ml jar of the whole yogurt (at room temperature) and pour it into a bowl, then add two jars of sugar and with a whisk start to work them together until you get a smooth cream. At this point, break the eggs and separate the egg whites and yolks in two separate bowls, then by activating the mixer again, add the yolks in the yogurt and sugar mixture until they are incorporated.

Still, with the mixer in action, add the oil evenly. Once it is well mixed, place a sieve directly on the bowl, pour the two jars of flour, the jar of starch, and finally the sachet of baking powder. Sift everything and always using the low-speed mixer, incorporate the powders, until a smooth and uniform compound is obtained. At this point, take the egg whites and beat them until stiff steaks.

Add them to your mixture in two or three times: start by adding a small number of egg whites and mix vigorously without fear of deflating the dough, then stir in the rest of the egg whites and mix gently with rotating movements from the bottom up, to avoid to disassemble the compound.

Once the dough of your cake is ready, grease and flour a round mold of 24 cm in diameter, then pour the mixture inside. At this point, bake the cake seven jars in a static oven preheated to 180 ° for 45 minutes; if the cake darkens on the surface, cover it with aluminum foil during the last 10 minutes of baking. You can check the cooking by testing the toothpick; once cooked, take it out of the oven and let it cool before turning it out and serving it.

## 2) Chiffon Cake
### Ingredients:

- **Sugar 300 g**
- **00 flour 290 g**
- **Water 200 g**
- **Sunflower oil 120 g**
- **Large eggs 6**
- **Vanilla bean 1**
- **Untreated lemon zest 1**
- **Sweet baking powder 1 sachet**
- **Salt up to 2 g**
- **Icing sugar to taste**

To prepare the chiffon cake, start sieving the yeast together with the flour in a bowl. Then add the sugar and salt. Stir to mix them in the best way. In another bowl, separate the yolks from the egg whites of 6 large eggs and set aside the egg whites. Add the water at room temperature and the seed oil to the yolks.

Then grate the rind of a lemon and cut into a vanilla bean and extract the seeds and add them to the yolk mixture. Beat the mixture with the whisk until a homogeneous mixture is obtained. Then add it to the dry ingredients (flour, sugar, and yeast), pouring it in one go.

Stir thoroughly with a whisk until creamy. Let this dough rest for a while and dedicate yourself to whipping the egg whites. Pour them into a bowl of a planetary mixer (if you do not have a planetary mixer, you can use an electric mixer), then activate the whisk and start whipping the egg whites when they have become foamy.

Once the egg whites are well whipped, transfer a part into the dough kept aside and mix quickly with a spatula to dilute the mixture. Then add the remaining egg whites a little at a time, always mixing with a spatula from top to bottom.

Now that the cake dough is ready, gently pour it into the chiffon cake mold: take a 22 cm diameter bottom mold, 26 cm surface diameter and 10 cm high. Try to distribute the dough evenly. Then bake the chiffon cake in a static oven preheated to 160 ° for about 60 minutes (for a 150 ° ventilated oven for 45-50 minutes), placing the cake in the lower part of the oven. Once cooked, take it out of the oven and let it cool.

When the chiffon cake has completely cooled, you will have to detach the upper part of the mold: you can help yourself with a thin and sharp knife. Your chiffon cake is ready to be sprinkled with icing sugar at will!

### 3) Stuffed peaches in the oven

**Ingredients:**

- **Medium, ripe and firm yellow peaches 800 g**
- **Dark chocolate 100 g**
- **Amaretti 80 g**

To prepare the stuffed peaches in the oven, start by rinsing and drying the peaches. Divide each peach in half and remove the core with a small knife. Also, dig a little the pulp around the hollow of the core and keep the peaches aside.

Now dedicate yourself to the filling: chop the pulp obtained from peaches and keep them aside. Take the chocolate, finely chop it and keep it aside. Take another bowl and crumble the macaroons inside in a coarse way. If you prefer, you can also chop them finely with the help of a mixer. Add the pulp of peaches to the crumbled amaretti.

Mix the ingredients and add the chocolate and mix. Fill the peaches with a few spoons of the filling, giving the filling the shape of a small dome. Finally, place the peaches in a lightly buttered baking dish close to each other, preferably without leaving any spaces. Bake in a static preheated oven at 180 ° C for 60 minutes (or in a fan oven at 160 ° C for 50 minutes). After the necessary time, take out the stuffed peaches and serve them to your guests while still hot!

### 4) Sweet made soon

**Ingredients:**

- **Sugar 200 g**
- **00 flour 220 g**
- **Butter 150 g**
- **Medium eggs 4**
- **Untreated lemon zest 1**
- **Vanilla bean 1**
- **Baking powder 8 g**

Start by placing the sugar and the softened butter into small pieces in a planetary mixer with whips and start working the mixture. Then take a stick of vanilla, cut it, take the seeds and add them to the mixture. Grate the lemon zest, then add the eggs to room temperature and whip them.

After mixing the mixture, sift the yeast and flour into a bowl, add it to the mixture and mix all the ingredients well, then stop the mixer. Grease and flour the mold of a donut with a diameter and begin to pour the mixture. Spread it with a spatula to distribute it evenly.

Bake the cake in a preheated static oven at 170 ° for 50 minutes or in a ventilated oven at 150 ° for about 40 minutes. Before baking, make sure that the cake is cooked by dipping a toothpick in it. If the toothpick is dry, it means that the cake is ready. Let the cake cool down early and complete the recipe with a sprinkling of icing sugar.

## 5) Fruit ice cream

### Ingredients:

- **Melon 1.2 kg**
- **Pineapple 2 kg**
- **Mango 600 g**
- **Strawberries 500 g**
- **Blackberries 500 g**

Start by cleaning the melon. Cut the ends of the melon and divide it in half. Remove the seeds that are inside; cut each half into not too thick slices, remove the peel from each slice and finally reduce them to cubes of about 2 cm thick.

Put the cubes in a tray being careful not to overlap them, cover with plastic wrap, and transfer to the freezer. When the fruit has hardened, you can transfer it to a frost bag for at least 12 hours. Now move on to cleaning the pineapple by removing the base and the tuft, then divide the pineapple into four parts, remove the wooden interior and remove the peel.

Divide each segment in half and cut the slices obtained into chunks of about 1 cm thick, then spread the pineapple on a tray, cover with plastic wrap and transfer it to the freezer: when the pineapple has hardened, always transfer it to a bag frost for at least 12 hours.

 As for cleaning the mango, remove the peel, then make cuts for a long time with the knife and separate the slices one at a time, until the core remains in your hand; cut each slice into cubes about 2 cm thick, spread them evenly on a tray, cover with plastic wrap and leave in the freezer for at least 12 hours. Now take care of the strawberries: wash and dry them, then remove the stalk and cut them in half; at this point, you can transfer them on a tray, without overlapping them, and leave them in the freezer to freeze for at least 12 hours.

Finally, wash and dry the blackberries gently and transfer them to a tray, leaving them whole, then place them in the freezer for at least 12 hours. When the fruit is frozen, you can blend it to create your refreshing dessert: pour the frozen melon into a blender or mixer equipped with steel blades and blend until it becomes creamy, then transfer it to a bowl.

In the same way, pour the frozen pineapple into the blender and blend until you get a creamy consistency; do the same thing with mango, with strawberries and frozen blackberries. Transfer your frozen fruit into separate bowls and serve immediately!

### 6) Sweet beetroot cake

### Ingredients:

- **Sugar 190 g**
- **00 flour 260 g**
- **Pre-cooked beets 400 g**
- **Dark chocolate 130 g**
- **Corn seed oil 230 g**
- **Eggs 3**
- **Baking powder for sweets 16 g**
- **Van pod**

We begin by removing the outer peel from the already cooked beets and diced. Then transfer them to the glass of the immersion mixer, stretch with a drizzle of oil (about 30 g, provided for the recipe), and blend. Keep the beet cream aside, and move on to the chocolate: coarsely chop it and dissolve it in a water bath.

When it is completely melted, keep it aside and let it cool. In the meantime, dedicate yourself to the dough. Place the sugar and eggs at room temperature in the mixer (you can also use an electric mixer) also add the seeds of a vanilla bean and activate the whisk.

Work the mixture until it is well frothy; then add the oil and continue working. Sift the flour with the baking powder and add them little by little to the dough. Lastly, add the chilled chocolate and continue to knead the dough for a few minutes so that it mixes perfectly. Now take the beetroot cream and add it to the dough stirring gently with a spatula until incorporated.

Then pour the dough into a 24 cm diameter cake tin previously buttered and lined with parchment paper. Bake in a preheated static oven at 170 ° for 65 minutes (or at 150 ° for 55 minutes if the oven is ventilated), and before baking, test the toothpick to check the cooking. Remove the cake from the oven; let it cool down. If you like, before serving your sweet beet cake, you can sprinkle icing sugar on the surface.

### 7) Sweet zucchini cake

**Ingredients:**

- **Zucchini 300 g**
- **00 flour 250 g**
- **Almond flour 100 g**
- **Eggs 3**
- **Corn seed oil 200 ml**
- **Sugar 250 g**
- **Sweet baking powder 1 sachet**
- **Vanilla bean**

To prepare the sweet zucchini cake, start by washing the zucchini, remove the ends and grate them in a large hole grater. Beat the whole eggs with the sugar until a foamy mixture is obtained, then add the 00 flour, the hazelnut (or almond) flour, the seeds of the vanilla pod, and the well-sifted yeast. Also, add the seed oil, mixing well, and finally the grated zucchini.

Mix well and pour the mixture into a 24/26 cm buttered and floured cake pan (or covered with parchment paper). Bake the courgette cake for about 60 minutes at 180 ° C, checking that it has been cooked with a toothpick. If it gets too dark on the surface after the first 40 minutes of cooking, cover it with aluminum foil. Let the zucchini cake cool before turning it out. Serve it sprinkled with icing sugar!

### 8)  Apple pie

#### Ingredients:

- **Apples (700 g clean) 930 g**
- **Sugar 200 g**
- **00 flour 250 g**
- **Butter 100 g**
- **Whole milk (at room temperature) 150 g**
- **Eggs (at room temperature) 2**
- **Lemons 1**
- **Baking powder for sweets 16 g**
- **Cinnamon powder ½ tsp**
- **Salt up to a pinch**

#### TO SPRAY
- **Icing sugar to taste**

To make the apple pie, first, melt the butter in a pendulum, and keep it aside. Grate the lemon zest and squeeze the juice to obtain about 30 g, then keep both the zest and the juice aside. Peel the apples and remove the core, then cut them into four parts and cut them into slices.

Put the sliced apples in a bowl and drizzle them with the lemon juice to prevent them from turning black. Then proceed to sift the 00 flour with the baking powder. Then, in a large bowl, pour the eggs and part of the sugar dose. Start whipping with the electric whisk and continue pouring the sugar little by little.

When the mixture starts to lighten, add a pinch of salt and continue whipping until you get a frothy dough. At this point, add the melted butter brought back to room temperature. Flavored with ground cinnamon and also add the grated lemon zest. Then continuing to whip with the whisk, add the sifted flour and baking powder a little at a time.

When the powders are completely incorporated, lower the speed of the electric whisks and pour the milk flush at room temperature.

When the milk is completely incorporated, stop the whips, the dough is ready. Now drain the apples in a colander to remove the lemon juice and pour them into the dough. Gently mix from bottom to top to incorporate them well. Grease and sprinkle a 22 cm diameter cake tin with sugar and pour the mixture. The cake is ready to be baked, bake it in a preheated static oven at 180 ° for about 55 minutes.

When cooked, take it out of the oven and let it cool. Sprinkle the cake with the icing sugar and serve

### 9) Paradise cake

**Ingredients:**

- **Light butter 170 g**
- **Icing sugar 170 g**
- **Sugar 40 g**
- **Salt up to 2,5 g**
- **Potato starch 70 g**
- **Sweet baking powder 3 g**
- **00 flour 100 g**
- **Vanilla bean**
- **Yolks 80 g**
- **Whole eggs 100 g**
- **½ lemon zest**
- **Orange peel ½**

**TO SPREAD THE CAKE**

- **Icing sugar to taste**

Start by sifting starch, flour, and yeast in a bowl and mix. In another bowl, put the butter into chunks, pour the pulp of half a vanilla bean and grate half the zest of lemon and orange. Start working with the electric whisk the vanilla-flavored butter, adding the icing sugar. When the mixture has assumed a soft and airy consistency, add the 80 g of yolks (about four medium egg yolks), then also pour in the salt and continue working the mixture with the electric whisk until a creamy consistency is obtained.

Keep aside and in another separate bowl pour the two whole eggs and add the granulated sugar; work everything with the electric whisk, and as soon as this mixture of eggs and sugar is frothy you can combine it with the one with butter, sugar, and yolks, alternating with the pouring of the powders. Then pour a little egg mixture, sugar, and mix well. Then add a part of the powders and continue mixing. Continue once more with the liquid part and finish with the powders until finished.

Take a 24 cm diameter mold and butter it, flour it and pour the dough of the paradise cake. Level it with until the surface is homogeneous. Bake the paradise cake in a static preheated oven at 170 ° for about 45-50 minutes (cover the cake with aluminum foil after 30 minutes of cooking if you see that it darkens excessively and continue cooking). Once ready (always try the toothpick), take it out of the oven and wait about 20 minutes before turning it upside down on a serving plate.

Remove the mold very gently and let it cool completely for about 1 hour. Once cold, sprinkle with icing sugar until a homogeneous layer is created on the surface. The cake is ready!

## 10) Yogurt soft cake

### Ingredients:

- **Low-fat yogurt 320 g**
- **Eggs (about 4) 220 g**
- **Room temperature butter 150 g**
- **Sugar 200 g**
- **00 flour 250 g**
- **Corn starch (cornstarch) 80 g**
- **Untreated lemon zest 1**
- **Salt up to a pinch**
- **Baking powder (1 sachet) 16 g**

To prepare the yogurt cake, cut the butter into cubes and let it soften. Then pour it into the bowl of a planetary mixer together with the sugar and start working it for at least 10 minutes. Once a creamy mixture is obtained, add the eggs one at a time, waiting for the previous one to be completely absorbed before adding the next.

Once you have incorporated all the eggs, add the yogurt and a pinch of salt, always with the whisk in action. Grate the zest of one lemon in the dough and mix gently with a spatula.

Add the flour in a bowl together with the yeast and corn starch, then sift them and pour them into the dough a little at a time. Mix well and gently with a spatula making a rotating movement from the bottom upwards in order not to disassemble the mixture.

Grease and flour a cake tin, then pour the mixture into it and level the surface with a spatula. Bake in a static preheated oven at 175 ° for about 50 minutes (if using the fan oven, cook 155 ° for 40 minutes). To test the correct baking of the cake, always try the toothpick. Once cooked, remove the cake from the oven and once it has cooled, remove it from the mold and leave it to cool completely. Your fluffy cake is ready to be enjoyed!

# Chapter 9: Recipes for snack

## 1) Tongues of cat

**Ingredients:**

- **Soft butter, ointment 50 g**
- **Icing sugar 60 g**
- **Egg whites 50 g**
- **Flour 0 50 g**

To prepare the cat's tongues, place the soft butter in a bowl. Add the icing sugar and mix with a spatula. In fact, this mass will not have to mount. Stir in the egg whites and stir again until creamy. Add the flour and stir again until a soft mass is obtained. Transfer the dough into a sac-à-poche with a 10 mm smooth nozzle.

Make sticks about 10 cm long on a dripping pan lined with parchment paper; you can make about 15 of them on the same dripping pan. Bake in a preheated convection oven at 190 ° for about 8 minutes. At this point, the cat's tongues will be ready. Remove from the oven and if you prefer to give a different shape than usual when they are still hot, transfer them to a rolling pin and let them cool. This way, you will get a wave shape. Otherwise, to obtain a straight shape, just let them cool in the pan. Transfer to a serving dish and serve or use them to make a dessert giving vent to your imagination.

## 2) Cookies with two ingredients

**Ingredients:**

- **Ripe bananas (approx. 2) 300 g**
- **Cereal muesli 100 g**
- **Dark chocolate chips (optional) to taste**

To make the biscuits with two ingredients, start by pouring the cereal muesli into a bowl, then peel the bananas, remove the filaments, and cut them into small pieces. Put the bananas in a potato masher and drop the puree obtained in the bowl with the muesli of cereals. Stir to mix the mixture, and then, if you like, add the chocolate drops. Stir again with the spoon to distribute the drops evenly, then take a dripping pan, cover it with parchment paper and distribute small piles of dough with a spoon, taking care to compact the biscuits well and space them apart to prevent sticking during cooking.

Leave the biscuits to rest in the freezer for 10 minutes, in this way they will be firmer and keep their shape well, then proceed by baking the biscuits in a preheated static oven for 15 minutes at 180 ° (in a convection oven at 160 ° for about 10 minutes). When cooked, take the biscuits out of the oven and, with the help of a spatula, gently remove them from the pan and transfer them to a wire rack to cool them. Your two-ingredient biscuits are ready to eat!

### 3) Cookies with chocolate chips

**Ingredients:**

- **Chocolate drops 100 g**
- **00 flour 500 g**
- **Eggs (medium) 2**
- **Brown sugar 200 g**
- **Vanilla bean 1**
- **Baking soda 3 g**
- **Salt up to a pinch**
- **Butter (softened) 180 g**

To make the chocolate chip cookies, start by placing the dark chocolate chips in the refrigerator so that we are very cold when you add them to the dough. Put the butter into pieces in a planetary mixer, pour the sugar and a pinch of salt, start kneading to obtain a cream. Incorporate the eggs and pour the sifted flour, then flavor with the vanilla bean seeds, add the baking soda mix the mixture, and lastly, add the very cold chocolate drops.

Now take the dough, give it the shape of a flat dough, wrap it with plastic wrap, and put it in the refrigerator for at least 30 minutes. After the rest time, resume the dough, divide it into small pieces, first give each one a spherical shape by turning them in your hands and then flatten them and create the typical teardrop shape. Transfer the biscuits to a tray lined with parchment paper and put them in the refrigerator for about 30 minutes, this will ensure that they keep their shape when baking.

Then proceed with the cooking: transfer the biscuits to a dripping pan lined with parchment paper and bake the biscuits in a preheated static oven at 180 ° for 15 minutes (or in a convection oven at 160 ° for 10 minutes). When cooked, take out the biscuits with chocolate chips and leave them to cool on a wire rack.

### 4)  Waffle

#### Ingredients:

- **00 flour 280 g**
- **Butter 220 g**
- **Medium eggs, at room temperature 6**
- **Baking powder for cakes 2 g**
- **Sugar 180 g**
- **Vanilla bean 1**
- **Salt up to 1 tsp**

#### TO SEAL

- **Fresh fruit to taste**
- **Maple syrup to taste**
- **Icing sugar to taste**

To prepare the waffles, melt the butter in a pendulum and let it cool. In the meantime, break the eggs at room temperature in a bowl and beat them lightly with a whisk, then add the sugar and mix again. Sift the yeast and flour directly into the bowl, add the salt and mix. Mix the powders well with the mixture and remove any lumps. Once it has cooled, pour the melted butter into the bowl little by little, so as to gradually incorporate it.

At this point, divide the vanilla pod and extract the seeds with the blade of a knife, add them to the mixture and mix again until a dense and homogeneous consistency is obtained. Cover the bowl with plastic wrap and let the dough rest in the refrigerator for an hour.

After the rest time, let the dough return to room temperature and, in the meantime, heat the waffle iron to bring it to temperature. When the plate is hot, brush it with a little melted butter and pour a ladle of dough into the honeycomb-shaped mold in order to completely cover the surface. Close the plate and cook for about 7-8 minutes (check the cooking status after 2.3 minutes))

When the waffles have taken on a beautiful golden color, open the lid, gently remove them from the plate and transfer them to a plate. Garnish the waffles as desired with maple syrup, fresh fruit and a shower of icing sugar.

### 5) Pralin almonds

#### Ingredients:

- **Almonds 150 g**
- **Sugar 120 g**
- **Water 35 g**

To make praline almonds, first, prepare a dripping pan lined with parchment paper. Now take a pan and pour the almonds, sugar, and water at room temperature inside.

Turn on the heat over medium-low heat and start mixing. In the beginning, the mixture of water and sugar will be very liquid, then it will start to boil and finally to crystallize, forming a patina around the almonds.

At this point, lower the heat slightly and continue stirring until the sugar starts to caramelize. Once browned, pour the almonds on the baking tray lined with parchment paper and space them apart; as they cool, divide them with your hands to prevent them from sticking together. Your praline almonds are ready to be enjoyed!

### 6) Candied ginger

**Ingredients:**

- **Water to taste**
- **Fresh ginger to clean 450 g**

   **FOR SECOND COOKING**

- **Boiled ginger 160 g**
- **Sugar 160 g**
- **Water 100 g**
- **Salt up to 1 tsp**
   **TO SEAL**

- **Sugar to taste**

Peel the ginger and then cut it into small pieces of about 2 cm. Place the ginger in a pan, pour over water until it is completely covered and boil it for about 30 minutes. Once boiled the ginger, drain it and place it in a saucepan, add the sugar100 g of water and salt.

Stir cook for 20 minutes over medium heat. After the cooking time, turn off the heat and let the mixture cool. Line a baking sheet with parchment paper and sprinkle the surface with sugar. Pour the cooled ginger, spread the pieces apart, and sprinkle with more sugar.

Collect the ginger in a foil to make the sugar adhere better. Let cool, and then you can put the candied ginger in a jar and enjoy it as a snack.

## 7)  Apple chips

### Ingredients:

- **Red Apples 500 g**
- **Sugar 150 g**
- **Water 200 g**
- **Lemon juice 1**

Start making the syrup by putting the sugar, water in a saucepan, and melt everything on low heat. Transfer the syrup obtained in a baking dish and let it cool; when it is at room temperature, squeeze a lemon and add its juice to the syrup. This will prevent the apples from blackening once sliced.

Wash the apples, remove the cores and slice them finely as if they were chips of chips (you can help yourself with a mandolin), obtaining a thickness of a couple of millimeters. Then dip the apple slices in the prepared syrup.

Drain them and place them on trays covered with parchment paper; put them to dry in a fan oven at 80 degrees for at least 5/6 hours, turning them with the help of a small knife halfway through drying. Probably, after cooking for 5/6 hours in the oven, the apple chips will still be soft to the touch, but don't worry; it's the effect of heat. As soon as they cool, they will become crunchy and ready to be nibbled!

## 8)  Spelled crackers

### Ingredients:

- **Spelled flour 250 g**
- **Dry white wine 80 g**
- **Extra virgin olive oil 50 g**
- **Cold butter butter 25 g**
- **Thyme 3 sprigs**
- **Salt up to 6 g**

## TO BRUSH AND CONDITION

- **Water to taste**
- **Coarse salt (optional) 8 g**
- **Poppy seeds 5 g**
- **Sunflower seeds 5 g**
- **Flax seeds 5 g**

To prepare the spelled crackers, start by pouring the spelled flour into a large bowl, add the fine salt, the fresh thyme and mix well. Add the butter and mix it with the flour mixture, then pour the olive oil, white wine and continue to work the mixture with your hands.

When the dough is compact, put it on a lightly floured work surface and roll it out with a rolling pin until you get a sheet of about 28x24 cm with a thickness of about 4-5 mm. Prick the dough with a fork and divide it into squares of about 4 cm on each side.

At this point, mix the coarse salt, poppy seeds, flax seeds, sunflower seeds in a small bowl and mix. Sprinkle the surface with the mix of seeds and coarse salt, pressing gently with your hands to make it stick.

Transfer the pastry squares to a dripping pan lined with parchment paper and brush them with a little water. Bake in a preheated static oven at 170 ° for about 25 minutes, in the middle shelf of the oven. Once cooked, let them cool, then the spelled crackers will be ready to be nibbled during the day!

## 9) Pasta balls with honey

Ingredients:

### FOR THE MIXTURE

- 250 g of 00 flour
- 4 g of baking powder
- 2 medium eggs
- 20 g of granulated sugar
- 30 g of melted butter
- Zest of half a lemon
- The zest of half an orange
- A pinch of salt

### TO DECORATE

- 150 g of honey
- 2 tablespoons of granulated sugar
- colored sprinkles

Prepare the dough to make the pasta balls in the oven by starting to sift the flour with the yeast. Add the other ingredients and mix until a compact and homogeneous paste is obtained. Now divide the dough into 5-6 portions and form with each of these portions a thin cylinder, with a diameter of about 1-2 cm. Cut the cylinders into pieces about 1 cm thick and arrange them on a large pan covered with slightly separated parchment paper. Let them rest in the refrigerator for 20 minutes.

Bake in a preheated oven at 180 ° for 10-11 minutes until the pasta has a golden color. In the meantime, heat the honey with the sugar in a saucepan. When the sugar is completely melted, pour the cooked pasta balls and candied fruit into the saucepan. Stir well until the biscuits are completely covered with honey and the rest. Put everything on a serving dish and let cool. Now they are ready to eat!

## 10) Biscuits with almonds

**Ingredients:**

- **2 eggs**
- **170 g of granulated sugar**
- **280 g of 00 flour**
- **½ teaspoon of baking soda**
- **40 g of soft butter**
- **70 g of shelled and unpeeled almonds**
- **1 tbsp honey**
- **1 yolk to brush**

To make the biscuits, start collecting the two whole eggs in a boule with granulated sugar and briefly work them with an electric mixer. Add the flour and baking soda and mix until a grainy dough is obtained. Add the butter, whole almonds, and honey. Knead the dough and make a dough.

Divide the dough into two parts and with the lightly floured hands obtained from each a loaf. Arrange them both on a baking sheet covered with parchment paper and brush them with the egg yolk. Bake in a preheated oven at 190 ° for 20 minutes. Withdraw them, let them rest for a few minutes, and cut each strand into diagonal slices, about a centimeter thick, thus obtaining biscuits. Brown the biscuits for another 5 minutes in the oven at 200 °.

Remove from the oven and let them cool down and they are ready to eat.

# Chapter 10: Drinks & Shakes

### 1) Golden milk

**Ingredients:**

- **Water 130 g**
- **Turmeric powder 40 g**
- **Black pepper 1 pinch**
- **FOR A GOLDEN MILK CUP**
- **Vegetable milk (almond or soy) 150 g**
- **honey 1 tbsp**

To prepare the golden milk, you have to start with turmeric paste. Pour the water in a saucepan together with a little pepper and bring to a boil. As soon as the water boils, turn off the heat and add the turmeric powder. Stir until you have a thick and grainy paste. Finally, transfer the turmeric paste to a jar in which you can store it. Now move on to the preparation of your cup of golden milk. In a saucepan, bring the vegetable milk to a boil and then transfer it to a jar and add a teaspoon of turmeric paste, then sweeten with honey and close the jar with the cap. Ready for your golden milk!

### 2) Banana milkshake

**Ingredients:**

- **Bananas 300 g**
- **Ice 60 g**
- **Cinnamon sticks 2 g**
- **Whole milk 150 g**

To prepare the banana smoothie, we start by cutting the bananas into chunks and inserting them in the mixer. Also, add the cinnamon, not too many ice cubes, and the milk at a standing temperature.

Operate the mixer until a thick and creamy mixture is obtained. Then pour it into the glasses and decorate with a few pieces of cinnamon. The milkshake is ready.

### 3) Yogurt smoothie

**Ingredients:**

- **Yogurt 250 g**
- **Lime juice (about 1) 13 g**
- **Pulp melon 420**
- **Pulp peaches 350**

Let's start by washing the peaches (it will take about 3), peel them, and remove them from the core, then cut them into coarse pieces and set them aside. Now the melon: cut it in half, remove the seeds and peel and cut it into pieces.

Cut the lime in half and squeeze it. Collect the juice obtained in a glass and keep it aside. Now take a blender and put the and melon. Pour the yogurt and lime juice, close the blender, and activate it. Keep blending until the mixture is creamy. Your yogurt smoothie is ready!

### 4) Almond milk

**Ingredients:**

- **Peeled almonds 200 g**
- **Water 1 l**
- **Acacia honey 85 g**

To prepare almond milk, first put the almonds in a bowl with 500 g of water for at least an hour to soak. After the hour, pour both the almonds and the water into a mixer, then add the remaining 500 g of water and honey. Blend everything until a homogeneous cream is obtained, then filter the mixture obtained through a narrow mesh strainer and refrigerate for at least an hour, covered with plastic wrap. Serve your almond milk cold or at room temperature.

### 5) Homemade tropical fruit juice

**Ingredients:**

- **450 g of pineapple**
- **250g mango**
- **2 oranges**
- **1 grapefruit**
- **1.2 liters of water**
- **100g of sugar**

Start by peeling the mango and cutting it into cubes. Peel the pineapple by cutting the ends first then in half and finally in four parts. Remove the central hard part and also make the cubes pineapple. After this, extract the juice of an orange and a grapefruit.

Now transfer the citrus juice and fruit cubes to the pot with water and sugar and cook for 15 minutes. Pass 15 minutes with a hand blender and whisk until you have a puree, and you will put them in sterilized glass jars. Close the jars and put them and put them in the refrigerator until the jars cool down. They are now ready to be tasted!

### 6) Non-alcoholic melon cocktail

**Ingredients:**

- **1 untreated lemon**
- **20 grams of sugar**
- **2 slices of melon**
- **2 slices of white melon**
- **400 milliliters of carbonated mineral water**

Rinse the lemon and peel without throwing away the zest. Divide the lemon in half, squeeze it, and filter the juice obtained by passing it in a colander. Put the filtered juice and the lemon zest in a saucepan together with 20 grams of sugar. Cook everything for 2 minutes on low heat, stirring.

Filter the syrup obtained and let it cool. Peel the melon and the white melon, remove the seeds and the white filaments. Cut the pulp of the melons into small pieces. Put the melon pieces in the blender until you have obtained a homogeneous mixture. Add the previously prepared syrup to the melon smoothie. Incorporate, little by little, the carbonated mineral water to your non-alcoholic cocktail.

 Blend again and put them in a container or cocktail glasses and put them in the refrigerator. Leave them to cool for a quarter of an hour. When finished, decorate the glasses as desired with straws and melon slices. Serve the non-alcoholic melon cocktail still very fresh.

### 7)  Smoothie cheesecake

**Ingredients:**

- **Lean cottage cheese 250 g**
- **Fresh liquid cream 250 g**
- **Icing sugar 30 g**
- **Strawberries 280 g**
- **Yellow peaches 380 g**

To make the cheesecake smoothie, first, wash the peach and strawberries, then peel the peach and cut it into pieces, transfer it to the mixer glass and blend to get a puree. Do the same operation with the strawberries, remove the green stalk, cut them into small pieces, and place in the mixer glass to blend them until you get a puree. Now pour the ricotta into a bowl, add ¾ of the fresh liquid cream, the icing sugar and blend everything with the immersion mixer to obtain a homogeneous cream. Now add the remaining fresh liquid cream and mix to mix.

Now make your own cheesecake smoothie. Use glasses of about 70 cl capacity. The smoothie is made up of a layer of ricotta cream alternated with fruit puree. Pour the first layer of cream, move the glass slightly between your hands to evenly distribute the first layer on the bottom, cover with peach or strawberry puree, then pour a layer of ricotta cream again and finish with the strawberry or peach puree. Serve your cheesecake smoothie fresh!

### 8) Apple cider

**Ingredients:**

- **700 grams of apples**
- **50 grams of sugar**
- **100 ml of water**
- **1 orange**
- **1 lemon**
- **2 cloves**
- **1 cinnamon stick**
- **1 fresh ginger**

To prepare the apple cider, start by cutting and squeezing the orange and obtaining the juice. Do the same with the lemon. Now wash, peel, and remove the core from the apples. At this point, cut the apples until they are cubed and put in the blender until the juice is obtained, then filter it with a strainer.

Now add the sugar and the orange and lemon juice and mix so as to mix all the flavors. Now add the fresh ginger, the cloves, the cinnamon, and cook for 10 minutes. Pass the 10 minutes and filter everything, and your apple cider is ready!

### 9) Chai latte

**Ingredients:**

- **200 ml milk**
- **200 ml water**
- **2 black tea bags**

- **1 pinch of cinnamon**
- **1 pinch of cardamom**
- **2 ginger sticks**
- **1 teaspoon maple syrup**

Start by putting the water in a saucepan and bring it to a boil. Once the water boils, turn off the stove and insert the tea bags and spices. After a couple of minutes, remove the tea bags and keep them brewing for another 4 minutes.

In the meantime, take another saucepan and pour milk and a teaspoon of maple syrup. With a wooden spoon, mix well until the syrup has completely drained. You can now add the infusion in the milk and mix well to mix the flavors. Ready!

### 10) Fruit and yogurt cocktails

**Ingredients:**

- **25 gr of strawberries**
- **25 gr of raspberries**
- **125 ml of cold milk**
- **125 ml of Cold Natural Yogurt**
- **1 Teaspoon Rose Water**
- **1/2 teaspoon of light honey**

To prepare it, put the milk, strawberries, raspberries, yogurt, rose water in the blender, and blend for about 30 seconds, mixing the ingredients well. Pour into a tall drink glass, mix and add the honey. Decorate with strawberry slices or a sprig of mint, serve immediately.

# Conclusion

GERD is a disorder related to the stomach and digestive system that creates irritation. The main reason behind this problem is poor nutrition, poor digestion, lack of sleep, and an incorrect lifestyle. Weight gain and other health complications can cause acid reflux. With GERD, heartburn is felt, and there is a feeling that food is coming back from the stomach.

The treatments to combat GERD in the initial phase is the correct intake of food, exercise, and following a healthy diet trying to reduce weight. If not treated well, it can cause further serious health complications such as cancer or ulcers. To get quick relief from GERD, you need to adopt some lifestyle changes such as taking small meals instead of full meals, following an exercise routine, reducing, limiting the intake of spicy and fried foods, and reducing. In the initial phase of GERD, it can be treated and prevented with healthy and organic food choices. Also, carry out an adequate medical check-up; this will help you find out how serious the problem is. Consult your family doctor and listen to his or her treatment recommendations and precautions. This is the first step you need to take to treat GERD. In this book, a series of healthy and organic recipes are mentioned that will help you finally enjoy good food and relief even in acid reflux conditions.

Made in the USA
Monee, IL
28 October 2020